Funded by
MISSION COLLEGE
Carl D. Perkins Vocational and Technical Education Act Grant

THE AIDS CONSPIRACY: SCIENCE FIGHTS BACK

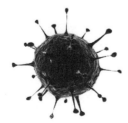

THE
AIDS
CONSPIRACY

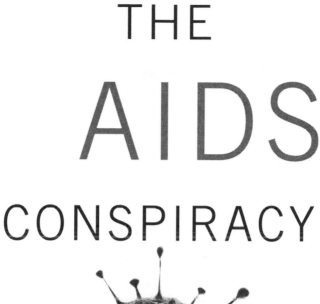

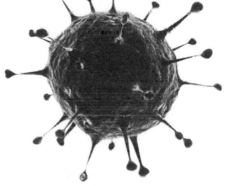

SCIENCE FIGHTS BACK

NICOLI NATTRASS

Columbia University Press

New York

COLUMBIA UNIVERSITY PRESS
Publishers Since 1893
New York   Chichester, West Sussex
cup.columbia.edu

Copyright © 2012 Columbia University Press

Library of Congress Cataloging-in-Publication Data
Nattrass, Nicoli.
    The AIDS conspiracy : science fights back / Nicoli Nattrass.
        p. ; cm.
    Includes bibliographical references and index.
    ISBN 978-0-231-14912-9 (cloth : alk. paper) —
    ISBN 978-0-231-52025-6 (ebook)
    I. Title.
    [DNLM: 1. HIV Infections—South Africa.   2. HIV Infections—
United States.   3. Acquired Immunodeficiency Syndrome—South
Africa.   4. Acquired Immunodeficiency Syndrome—United States.
5. Health Policy—South Africa.   6. Health Policy—United States.
7. Public Opinion—South Africa.   8. Public Opinion—United States.
WC 503]
362.196'9792—dc23

                                                              2011045297

∞

Columbia University Press books are printed on permanent and
durable acid-free paper.
This book is printed on paper with recycled content.
Printed in the United States of America

c 10 9 8 7 6 5 4 3 2 1

Designed by Lisa Hamm

FOR DAVID GILBERT

CONTENTS

ACKNOWLEDGMENTS

I would like to thank Harry Collins, Patrick Fitzgerald, David Gilbert, Eduard Grebe, John Moore, Clara Rubincam, Jeremy Seekings, and two anonymous reviewers for their helpful comments on earlier drafts. Thanks also to Roy Thomas for his excellent editing.

THE AIDS CONSPIRACY: SCIENCE FIGHTS BACK

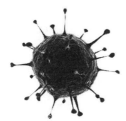

1

THE CONSPIRATORIAL
MOVE AGAINST HIV SCIENCE
AND ITS CONSEQUENCES

Most people do not believe conspiracy theories about the acquired immune deficiency syndrome (AIDS). But suspicions that the human immunodeficiency virus (HIV) may have been created in a laboratory, and that the pharmaceutical industry invented AIDS as a means of selling toxic drugs, persist on both sides of the Atlantic. During the 2008 US presidential campaign, Barack Obama had to deal with politically embarrassing revelations that his pastor, Jeremiah Wright, believed the government had created HIV to harm blacks.[1] Four years earlier, the Nobel Prize–winning Kenyan ecologist Wangari Maathai stunned the world with her casual observation that HIV had been "created by a scientist for biological warfare."[2] Most tragically, conspiracy theories about HIV were promoted in the early 2000s by then South African president Thabo Mbeki and his health minister Manto Tshabalala-Msimang—with devastating consequences for AIDS policy.

AIDS conspiracy theories range from the claim that the HIV is a man-made bioweapon, to the "AIDS denialist" assertions that HIV is harmless and antiretroviral drugs themselves cause AIDS. Although very different,

both theories make a "conspiratorial move" against HIV science by implying that scientists and clinicians have either been duped by, or are part of,
a broader conspiracy to inflict harm. This, in turn, undermines trust in the
scientific consensus on HIV prevention and treatment. A growing body
of research shows that AIDS conspiracy beliefs in the United States and
South Africa are associated with risky sex,[3] with not adhering to antiretroviral treatment,[4] and with not testing for HIV.[5]

My interest in AIDS conspiracy theory was born in 1999–2000 when
Mbeki questioned HIV science and claimed that the pharmaceutical industry was conspiring with the US government to inflict toxic drugs on
Africans. He and Tshabalala-Msimang consequently delayed the use of
antiretrovirals for both HIV prevention and treatment—causing literally
hundreds of thousands of unnecessary deaths from AIDS (see chapter 5).
But the harm to public health was more insidious than this. By casting
aspersions on medical science itself, a healing vacuum was created into
which rushed alternative healers of all descriptions. The resulting confusion was reinforced by an international group of self-styled HIV "dissident"
thinkers, some of whom were also associated with promoting alternative
therapies. Contesting them (including as a founding member of the anti–
AIDS-denial website www.aidstruth.org) was a painful lesson in the difficulties involved in countering the conspiratorial move against HIV science.
This book is the product of my attempts to understand the nature of AIDS
conspiracy beliefs, why they matter, and how to challenge them.

CONSPIRACY THEORY, SKEPTICISM, AND THE CONSPIRATORIAL MOVE

The term *conspiracy theory* is pejorative in that it implies irrationality and implausibility. Its use here is not to suggest that the very idea of a conspiracy is
irrational or implausible. Indeed, the origins of the "HIV as US bioweapon"
theory can be traced to a real-world conspiracy between Soviet and East
German intelligence operatives to spread misinformation (see chapter 2).
Furthermore, if a medical conspiracy is understood loosely as an agreement

between researchers to act in a way that harms others, then the infamous Tuskegee Study conducted between 1932 and 1972, which left syphilis patients untreated in order to observe the natural progression of the disease, and the more recent Vioxx scandal, in which the reporting period for heart attacks during the clinical trial was deliberately shortened to conceal these side-effects, could both reasonably be seen as "conspiracies."[6] Given the potential for the profit motive to undermine scientific integrity, there are good grounds for skepticism toward the pharmaceutical industry in general and industry-sponsored clinical trials in particular. But when this skeptical stance morphs into an *a priori* certainty that an entire body of science and related clinical practice has been corrupted and that none of the evidence it generates can be trusted, then a fundamental conspiratorial move is made. A conspiracy theory is thus born which is implausible in scope (it implies an international plot involving corporations, governments, scientists, and physicians that is so secret and cunning that hundreds of thousands have been conned into believing lies) and irrefutable in character.

Some scholars argue that even though conspiracy theories may be implausible and irrefutable, they are nevertheless logically possible and thus cannot be rejected out of hand.[7] But, as philosopher Brian Keeley observes, "there is much in the world that is possible but nonetheless is literally incredible."[8] Plausibility, credibility, and judgment all ought to matter in coming to "some consensus as to when belief in the theory entails more scepticism than we can stomach."[9] A key contention of this book is that the conspiratorial move against HIV science is "incredible" given the substantial evidence that antiretrovirals reduce HIV transmission and AIDS mortality. HIV scientists, pro-science advocates, and AIDS treatment activists find the conspiratorial move hard to stomach for another reason: that it encourages people to reject HIV prevention and treatment messages. Their contestation with proponents of AIDS conspiracy theories forms a second, central theme of the text.

Rejecting medical science poses an obvious problem: how are illnesses to be addressed in its absence? Some seek answers in what Colin Campbell termed the "cultic milieu," i.e., that fluid countercultural space in which alternative therapies and conspiracy theories flourish.[10] Ironically, many of those seeking alternatives to biomedicine render themselves vulnerable to what I term "cultropreneurs," i.e., those who both promote conspiracy theories about Western medicine while offering seemingly safer (more "natural" or "holistic") alternatives in its place. Pro-science advocates have responded by exposing the claims of cultropreneurs as unsubstantiated (if not fraudulent) and promoting evidence-based medicine.

CONTESTING AIDS CONSPIRACY THEORY

The history of racialized medical abuse and biowarfare in South Africa and the United States provides a fertile social terrain for AIDS conspiracy theories to take root. But when they are promoted by leaders, they gain additional purchase in the public imagination. Thus in 2000, when Tshabalala-Msimang circulated the "HIV as US bioweapon" conspiracy theories of William Cooper—a white right-wing militia leader from Arizona—she not only extended his audience into Africa, but legitimized his claims precisely because she was health minister.

Incongruous though it may seem to have an African cabinet minister promoting the views of a white American militiaman, this kind of borrowing of ideas from seemingly incompatible sources is common in the cultic milieu. But precisely because of the political incongruity of such connections, AIDS treatment activists have been able to use it as a lever to contest AIDS conspiracy beliefs. Thus, when controversial US expatriate physician William Campbell Douglass promoted a version of the Soviet–East German story about HIV being a US bioweapon, David Gilbert (a leftist prisoner in the United States) was able to counter its influence in the African-American community by exposing not only the scientific and other weaknesses in Douglass's argument but also his anti–civil rights record.

Credibility is also at stake in the battle over AIDS denialism. When President Mbeki appointed Peter Duesberg, the Californian-based virologist and leading proponent of AIDS denialism, to his "Presidential AIDS Advisory Panel" in 2000, he boosted Duesberg's status and profile. But in so doing, he also turned himself and Duesberg into targets for counterattacks by HIV scientists and AIDS activists.

Unlike the AIDS origin conspiracy theorists, Duesberg is an academic with a creditable scientific research record, though not on HIV or AIDS. But because of his scientific standing in other areas (cancer research), he provides a patina of scientific legitimacy to AIDS denialist claims. This has helped bolster the organized AIDS denialist movement and given it a tangible social presence. Conspiracy narratives serve organizational as well as ideological functions for this movement. Depicting Duesberg as a latter-day Galileo persecuted by a venal "AIDS establishment" serves to reinforce social solidarity by presenting his supporters with the thrilling identity of being in receipt of "the truth," and as brave whistle-blowers standing up for "real" scientific progress. In a somewhat cultish manner, Duesberg is their "hero scientist" who both constructs and legitimizes their denial that HIV is harmful and that antiretroviral treatments work. But his message gains added power by a second, important pillar of AIDS denialism: the messages of hope and (false) promises of the cultropreneurs who also populate the movement.

AIDS denialist cultropreneurs use Duesberg's theories to cast aspersions on HIV as the cause of AIDS. Instead, they attribute AIDS to the "stress" of an HIV-positive diagnosis, to "toxic" antiretroviral drugs, poor nutrition, and recreational drug abuse. Predictably, they offer a range of alternative therapies and products to deal with such immune deficiency. But because none of these has been (scientifically) proven to work, a further symbolic role has emerged: that of "living icon"—people who, literally, put their HIV-positive bodies on the line by supposedly demonstrating that they can live safely and healthily using alternative therapies. Christine Maggiore, the now deceased HIV-positive mother who refused to take precautions against infecting her children with HIV, was for a long time the central living icon—despite losing her three-year-old daughter in 2005 from what the coroner determined to be AIDS. Sympathetic, praise-singing journalists and filmmakers serve a further important organizational function by taking the messages and stories of the hero scientists and living icons to the general public.

These roles of hero scientist, living icon, cultropreneur, and praise-singer are evident in another organized challenge to mainstream medical science—notably the anti-vaccination lobby where Andrew Wakefield (a doctor who claimed the mumps, measles, rubella [MMR] vaccine caused autism and was later struck off the medical roll in the UK for unethical research practices) functions as both hero scientist and provider of alternative therapies for autism. Like AIDS denialism, the anti-vaccination movement offers supporters an oppositional identity of being part of an enlightened minority, seeking alternative cures while standing up to a corrupt scientific establishment bent on concealing or refusing to investigate the truth. These similarities are touched on in the concluding chapter, which contextualizes the fight against AIDS conspiracy theory within the broader contemporary struggle for evidence-based medicine.

Conspiracy theories which cast suspicion on medical science itself are particularly pernicious. Not only are cultropreneurs incentivized to promote them, but they are able to tap into a large audience by offering natural-sounding alternative therapies and new forms of identity. But precisely because the conspiratorial move against science can seriously undermine public health, growing numbers of pro-science activists are contesting it and promoting the cause of science and reason in the public sphere.

OUTLINE OF THE BOOK

Chapter 2 opens the analysis by exploring the nature and prevalence of AIDS origin conspiracy beliefs. The Soviet–East German misinformation campaign is touched on as the origin of the "HIV as US bioweapon" conspiracy theory, but most attention is paid to the history of medical abuse and biowarfare that gives the story such social traction in the United States and South Africa. The chapter also touches on the origin of HIV in Africa, and the early counter-narrative that HIV was injected into the African population by vaccination programs. The key argument is that AIDS origin conspiracy theories resonate with, and are shaped by, the local historical context—but that the role played by key individuals in constructing and promoting these ideas is also a crucial part of the story.

Explaining AIDS origin conspiracy beliefs with reference only to contextual factors cannot account for the fact that most people do not endorse them. Chapter 3 takes up this issue by exploring the individual determinants of such beliefs, using survey data on young adults in Cape Town. The results suggest that psychological factors matter, but so do political preferences, attitudes, and socioeconomic location. Notably, people who trusted Tshabalala-Msimang more than her successor as health minister were more likely to believe conspiracy theories about the origin of HIV—as were those who had never heard of the Treatment Action Campaign, the civil society organization that opposed Mbeki on AIDS.

This poses the tricky problem of how to assess the role of leaders in promoting AIDS conspiracy theories. While it is important to understand the social and historical context for AIDS conspiracy beliefs, analytical space needs to be maintained for critiquing leaders when they promote or endorse them. When Mbeki and Tshabalala-Msimang blocked the use of antiretrovirals, they rendered their already-vulnerable followers even more vulnerable. Likewise, when Louis Farrakhan, the charismatic leader of the Nation of Islam in the United States, promoted AIDS conspiracy theories while offering an ineffective "cure" in its place, an already-vulnerable population was rendered even more so. The book discusses both these examples of poor leadership (chapters 5 and 3, respectively).

Chapter 4 concludes the discussion of AIDS origin conspiracy theory by exploring the way it has been contested by David Gilbert. It also discusses a postmodern critique of Gilbert, and his response to it. The chapter provides a forum for engaging with relativist arguments that since we cannot "know" that AIDS conspiracy theories are false, contesting them is ultimately a rhetorical strategy entailing the assertion of one form of knowledge over another. I argue that reason and judgment can and should be brought to bear on the issue and that contesting AIDS conspiracy theory in a way that is sensitive to the political credibility of scientific evidence is helpful.

The rest of the book focuses on AIDS denialism and the conspiratorial move it makes against HIV science. Chapter 5 explores the relationship between scientific expertise and political leadership through the lens of AIDS policy in South Africa under Mbeki. It argues that Mbeki's attempt to facilitate a scientific debate was inappropriate—as policymaker, he should have bowed to expertise. In reviewing the role of AIDS denialism, the chapter also poses the question why Mbeki went down this road.

Various explanations are considered, but in the end the answer is uncertain. What we do know is that he refused to accept the legitimacy or authority of HIV science and, like Duesberg and his supporters, was impervious to the evidence for the efficacy of antiretroviral treatment. He seems, in other words, to have made the conspiratorial move against HIV science at a fundamental level—and one characteristic of the AIDS denialist community.

Chapter 6 considers the key elements of organized AIDS denialism, showing that social and symbolic factors are powerfully at work. It argues that the key players are a closely knit group, serving as board members in each other's organizations, and that the four symbolically and ideologically powerful roles described earlier (hero scientist, cultropreneur, living icon, and praise-singer) are evident. But precisely because these roles are so important, those filling them have become targets for the rival virtual communities that have formed in response to AIDS denialism. As discussed in the chapter, various websites and blogging activities are dedicated to exposing AIDS denialist myths and to discrediting the key players.

Chapter 7 focuses on how the scientific community has challenged Duesberg's claims about HIV pathogenesis and treatment. This ranges from published rebuttals of his claims to, more recently, taking direct action against a journal for publishing, without first subjecting it to peer review, a paper by Duesberg defending Mbeki's stance on AIDS. The incident is interesting not only for what it tells us about how and why scientists feel compelled to defend scientific practices, in this case peer review, but also about the importance of context—the unnecessary deaths in South Africa—which shaped the moral indignation behind the actions. It shows that the defense of science can be driven by normative considerations and that civil society as well as the scientific community engages in it.

Chapter 8 concludes the book by drawing parallels between the AIDS denialist movement and another example of organized opposition to medical science which employs the same conspiratorial moves and symbolic roles of AIDS denialism: the anti-vaccination movement. In an interesting parallel, poor political leadership also boosted skepticism toward vaccines in 2002 when then UK prime minister Tony Blair equivocated over whether his son had been vaccinated or not—while the press published stories about his wife's support for alternative and mystical therapies.

Chapter 8 ends with a reflection on how pro-science advocates are defending medical science in the public sphere, especially on the Internet. This includes setting up dedicated websites exposing cultropreneurs as "quacks," posting critiques of pseudoscientific and mystical claims, and engaging in debates through comment threads and blogs. While some analysts worry that the Internet is allowing people to cocoon themselves in rival thought communities (in that people can select what they want to read and hear), it is nevertheless the case that substantial space exists for contestation on the Internet. Science may be "under siege," as a recent collection of essays was titled,[11] but there is a guerrilla force gaining strength in the blogosphere, in newspaper columns and popular books. On a somewhat optimistic note, the book concludes that this modern manifestation of the enlightenment project in defense of science and reason is alive and well.

2

AIDS ORIGIN CONSPIRACY THEORIES
IN THE UNITED STATES AND SOUTH AFRICA

HIV is genetically very similar to the Simian immunodeficiency virus (SIV) in primates, and there is strong scientific evidence that different varieties of HIV evolved
in humans after several strains of SIV crossed the species
barrier at different points (see pp. 28–31). Yet a small but significant number
of people in the United States and South Africa believe that HIV/AIDS is
man-made, possibly with genocidal intent.

Social scientists agree that historical and contextual factors are crucial in
understanding why these claims resonate for many, especially black, people.
These include the infamous Tuskegee Study, and the history of bioweapon
research and testing in the United States and South Africa. This chapter
argues that these are indeed important historical roots for suspicion, but
that understanding how conspiracy theories are shaped and propagated by
key players is also important. That AIDS origin conspiracy beliefs reflect
local concerns yet span racial, political, and national boundaries speaks to
a more fluid and complex situation than a simple "there are good historical
reasons for these beliefs" analysis might suggest.

The chapter begins with a discussion of the empirical evidence for the extent of AIDS origin conspiracy beliefs in the United States and South Africa (the only countries for which survey data exist) and then explores the South African "ecotype" in more depth, pointing also to the role of imported ideas. The chapter then turns to a discussion of the origin of the "HIV as US bioweapon" myth (Soviet and East German propaganda), suspicions that HIV may have been transmitted through contaminated vaccines, and scientific evidence as to why this is not the case. It concludes with a discussion of why AIDS origin conspiracy theories are thinkable given the historical context of racialized suspicion of government and medical practice in the United States.

RACE AND THE PREVALENCE OF AIDS ORIGIN CONSPIRACY BELIEFS

Belief in AIDS origin conspiracy theories is highly racialized in the United States. As early as 1990, a *New York Times*/CBS poll found that 10 percent of black New Yorkers believed that it was true that "the virus that causes AIDS was deliberately created in a laboratory in order to infect black people," and a further 19 percent thought it may be true—whereas the numbers for white New Yorkers were 1 percent and 5 percent, respectively.[1] Higher levels of AIDS conspiracy beliefs among African-Americans were subsequently found among US college students and in the general population in New Jersey, Texas, and Florida.[2] Surveys at Gay Pride events in Michigan, California, and Maryland also showed higher levels of AIDS conspiracy beliefs among black respondents—as did a survey among AIDS patients in Texas.[3] These various surveys are summarized in table 2.1.

A similar pattern appears to be the case in South Africa. According to a 2009 survey of young adults in Cape Town, 16 percent of black respondents agreed that "AIDS was invented to kill black people" and that "AIDS was created by scientists in America" (whereas only 1 percent and 3 percent of other people, respectively, agreed with those statements). These levels of endorsement of AIDS conspiracy beliefs (discussed further in chapter 3) are

TABLE 2.1

AIDS CONSPIRACY BELIEFS AMONG AFRICAN-AMERICANS

QUESTION AND YEAR OF STUDY	SAMPLE	AGREE
MAN-MADE ORIGINS OF HIV		
AIDS is a man-made virus (1990)	1,056 churchgoers in 5 US cities[g]	34%
HIV is a man-made virus (2001)	US sample: 71 adults aged 18-45[e]	50%
HIV is a man-made virus (2002–2003)	US sample: 500 adults aged 15-44[f]	48%
HIV is a man-made virus (2004)	239 men at US Gay Pride events[k]	50%
AIDS was started by an experiment that went wrong (1997-98)	1,546 people assisting in a program for drug addicts, Baltimore[b]	45%
AIDS was produced in a government laboratory (2002–2003)	US sample: 500 adults aged 15–44[f]	27%
HIV is a man-made virus (2008)	181 patients on antiretroviral treatment	52%
AIDS was produced in a government laboratory (2008) in Los Angeles[j]		46%
There is some truth in reports that the AIDS virus was produced in a germ warfare laboratory (1988)	941 college students, Washington, D.C.[a]	38%
GENOCIDAL ORIGINS OF HIV		
AIDS is a form of genocide against the black race (1990)	979 churchgoers in 5 US cities[c]	35%
AIDS is a form of genocide against the black race (1990)	800 Households in Maryland[a]	15%
AIDS was deliberately created in a laboratory order to infect black people (1990)	408 New Yorkers (10% said it was true, 19% in said it might be true)[n]	10%
The government deliberately spread the AIDS virus in the black community (1992)	Phone survey, New Jersey, 74 respondents[g]	31%
AIDS is intended to wipe blacks off the face of the earth (1996)	715 black parishioners of 35 Louisiana churches[h]	27%
The AIDS virus was deliberately created to infect black people (1998)	91 northeastern college students[i]	60%
AIDS was created to kill blacks and poor folks (1997–98)	1,546 people assisting in a program for drug addicts, Baltimore[b]	25%

TABLE 2.1 *(CONTINUED)*

QUESTION AND YEAR OF STUDY	SAMPLE	AGREE
GENOCIDAL ORIGINS OF HIV *(CONTINUED)*		
AIDS is an agent of genocide created by the United States government to kill off minority populations (1997–98)	441 respondents in Houston shopping malls[c]	29%
HIV/AIDS is a man-made virus that the federal government made to kill and wipe out black people (1999)	520 households in San Bernardino County[d]	27%
I believe that AIDS is intended to wipe blacks off the face of the earth (2004)	170 locally elected officials in Louisiana[l]	30%
AIDS is a form of genocide against African-Americans (2001)	US sample: 71 adults aged 18–45[e]	26%
AIDS was created by the government to control the African-American population (2001)		23%
The government is using AIDS as a way of killing off minority groups (2001)	422 HIV-positive people in care in the deep South[o]	23%
AIDS was created and spread by the CIA (2002–2003)	US sample: 500 adults aged 15–44[f]	12%
AIDS is a form of genocide against blacks (2002–2003)		15%
AIDS was created by the government to control the black population (2002–2003)		16%
AIDS was created by the government to control the black population (2008)	181 patients on antiretroviral treatment in Los Angeles[j]	42%
AIDS is a form of genocide, or planned destruction, against blacks (2008)		40%
HIV was created and spread by the CIA (2008)		28%
The government is using AIDS as a way of killing off minority groups (2009)	555 Florida residents aged 18–39 (phone survey)[m]	24%

Sources: [a]Thomas and Quinn (1993:332–33); [b]Bohnert and Latkin (2009:761); [c]Ross, Essien, and Torres (2006:343); [d]Klonoff and Landrine (1999:455); [e]Bogart and Bird (2003:1062); [f]Bogart and Thorburn (2005:215); [g]Thomas and Quinn (1991:1499); [h]Parsons et al. (1999:212); [i]Crocker et al. (1999:946); [j]Bogart, Galvan et al. (2010); [k]Hutchinson et al. (2007:604); [l]Simmons and Parsons (2005:591); [m]Darrow, Montanea, and Gladwin (2009); [n]DeParle (1990); [o]Whetten et al. (2006:718).

significant, but lower than that reported in other less representative studies in South Africa[4] and the United States.

That black people are most likely to agree with these conspiratorial accounts is particularly worrying given that the HIV epidemic is especially virulent in the black populations of both countries. As of 2006 (the most recent US estimates) HIV prevalence among African-Americans was 1.7 percent, i.e., eight times higher than that for the rest of the population.[5] As shown in figure 2.1, HIV prevalence in South Africa is much higher overall, but similarly skewed toward the (black) African population.

Why does a significant minority of people in the United States and South Africa endorse survey statements about HIV being deliberately manufactured to cause harm—and why are there strong racial dimensions to these beliefs? In addressing this issue, it is useful to break it down into a subset of questions probing the context for these beliefs: why is the "AIDS as US bioweapon" story global in its reach; what makes the story thinkable both in South Africa and the United States; and what are the roots of racialized suspicion?

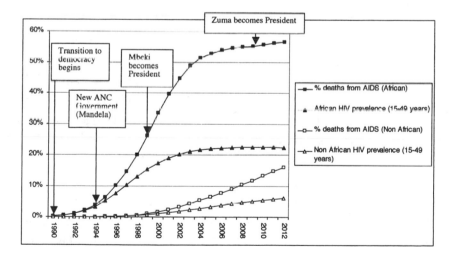

FIGURE 2.1 HIV prevalence and AIDS deaths in South Africa (author's projections using the ASSA2003 model, which can be downloaded from http://aids.actuarialsociety.org.za/ASSA2003-Model-3165.htm).

GLOBAL AIDS ORIGIN CONSPIRACY THEORY
AND THE SOUTH AFRICAN ECOTYPE

Other deadly epidemics, notably cholera, have sparked conspiracy theories,[6] and vaccine conspiracy theories regularly cross international boundaries.[7] Yet AIDS origin conspiracy theories appear to be uniquely global in their reach, no doubt reflecting both the scale of the epidemic (at least 25 million deaths from AIDS worldwide have occurred since 1980) and the accompanying fear and stigma. They have been reported around the world from the earliest days of the epidemic[8] and, as cultural theorist Paula Treichler observers, "circulate geographically with astonishing ease, serving as templates readily adapted to the charged social divisions and power inequalities of the epidemic's latest home."[9]

The idea that AIDS conspiracy theories travel easily while adapting to local conditions is consistent with what scholars of urban legends call "ecotypification."[10] In this approach, contemporary legends have two "anchors," a "legend kernel that remains constant across social situations" and the "details of ecotypification" rooted in local settings.[11] Local ecotypes of AIDS conspiracy theories have been recorded in Zimbabwe[12] and South Africa. The earliest recorded South African theory (dating from the late 1980s) claims that it was Israeli scientists working with racist white South Africans who manufactured and spread HIV.[13] That particular ecotype reflects the close alliance at the time between Israel and the apartheid government. However, by the 2000s, the most popular story appears to be that HIV had been invented by American scientists and/or the US Central Intelligence Agency (CIA), possibly in collaboration with Wouter Basson, the head of the apartheid government's chemical and biological weapons program.[14] Basson, who came to be known as "Dr. Death" was tried in a highly publicized case for manufacturing harmful substances for use against liberation forces.[15] As journalists Marléne Berger and Chandré Gould note, the trial, which lasted over thirty months, was a "tale of subterfuge and sophistry, politics and power, murder and mad science."[16] It is thus unsurprising that AIDS conspiracy stories evolved to incorporate him into the frame.

Basson was a cardiologist who headed the South African Defence Force chemical and biological warfare program from 1980 to 1992. Known as Project Coast, this program first came to light in 1998 in an amnesty application before the South African Truth and Reconciliation Commission. Subsequent investigative journalism revealed that his program included various wide-ranging projects, from attempting to breed a "super-wolf dog," to developing a contraceptive aimed specifically at the black population, to the search for the "ultimate murder weapon" that would be undetectable in autopsies.[17] These findings led to Basson's being charged on multiple counts of murder.

During Basson's trial, further innovative poisons and killing mechanisms were reported to have been used, and even spread to the United States and Britain. As one press report put it:

> For the men in white coats toiling over their test-tubes, there was, it seems, no limit to their perverse imaginations as they built a bizarre arsenal of murder weapons. These included anthrax, the heavy-metal poison thallium and cyanide being planted in the gum of envelopes, dusted on cigarette tips and put into chocolates. Colourless, odourless and tasteless, thallium causes an effect easily mistaken for a brain haemorrhage. Everyday items vitamin pills, orange juice, sugar, whisky were poisoned. Bottles of cholera organisms were issued to members of the special security forces to contaminate water supplies. Umbrellas and walking sticks concealed poison injectors, syringes were disguised as screwdrivers, and rings were made with hidden compartments for poison.[18]

Even underpants were poisoned—as was the case with Frank Chikane, an anti-apartheid leader and subsequent right-hand man to President Nelson Mandela—who, fortunately, survived the assault. Witnesses told of how "enemies" (predominantly black men suspected of being anti-apartheid fighters) were sedated and killed with experimental poisons and injections, and how "vast" quantities of narcotics were manufactured, supposedly for "crowd control."[19] Witnesses also revealed how combatants from Namibia had been tranquilized with darts and then thrown into the sea

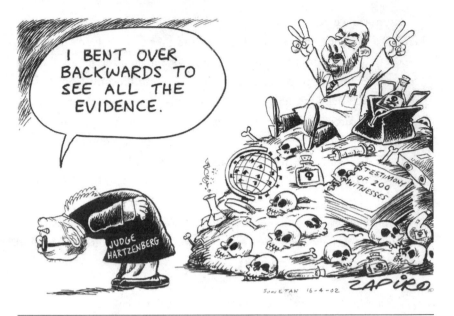

FIGURE 2.2 Public commentary on the acquittal of Wouter Basson (cartoon by Zapiro, Apr. 16, 2002, in *The Sowetan*, Johannesburg). © Zapiro. Reprinted with permission.

from helicopters. After a long trial, Basson was eventually acquitted by an elderly white judge, who ruled that insufficient evidence had been provided to link him directly to actual murders. But the fact of the atrocities, which had been accepted as such by the Truth and Reconciliation Commission, reverberated through the popular culture. The cartoon depicted in figure 2.2 sums up a broad feeling that justice had not been well served.

In their ethnographic research, Isak Niehaus and Gunvor Jonsson recorded many different stories circulating in African communities about the way in which Basson supposedly contributed to the spread of AIDS. Most of these reflect the information that came out of the Basson trial and speak to the history of the liberation struggle that was waged by the African National Congress (ANC) in South Africa:

> Allegedly, Dr Basson distributed HIV by various means. He put it in the
> food, water reservoirs, and clothes of black people; in the injections given

to hospital patients; in TB and smallpox vaccines; and even in the free, government-distributed condoms. However, most informants saw black soldiers as the prime agents for transmitting HIV. Dr Basson allegedly placed the virus in the rivers from which soldiers of the ANC's military wing, Umkhonto We Sizwe (MK) drank, and he laced the malaria tablets given to black South African Defence Force soldiers with HIV. Dr Basson purposefully created a slow virus so that the soldiers could spread it to as many women as possible.[20]

But the fact that "the Americans" and "the CIA" (sometimes, but not always, working with Basson) also feature strongly in the South African eco-type is worthy of consideration. From the early days of the HIV epidemic in South Africa, African suspicions about the intentions of whites and "the Americans" have been evident. Political sociologist Adam Ashforth notes that by the late 1980s the apartheid government recognized that HIV was spreading in the general African population and began to provide free condoms in clinics and to promote AIDS awareness campaigns—but that these were seen as an attempt to secure white domination by reducing the black birthrate: "having never buried anyone from a disease named AIDS they doubted the reality of the condition, jokingly referring to AIDS as standing for 'American Invention to Discourage Sex.'"[21] The link between "Americans" and racist whites surfaced again in the Basson trial, with Basson himself claiming that the British and the Americans were cooperating with him in return for information about chemical weapons used by Soviet-backed African countries.[22] So, the idea that the apartheid government had been collaborating with the United States was certainly "in the air." Even so, the post-apartheid context is important too, as the meaning of "the Americans" and "the CIA" would have had a different ring to it under a majority African government than would have been the case during the apartheid period when Basson and his henchmen were in power.

South Africa made the transition to democracy in 1994, and since then the ANC has governed the country. Whites continue to be blamed in many popular narratives for the spread of HIV—but through non-state vehicles such as farmers supposedly injecting fruit with contaminated blood, or medical professionals deliberately injecting people with it.[23] In some accounts, the sharp rise in HIV prevalence and AIDS deaths soon after the transition to democracy (fig. 2.1) has been linked to white anger and jealousy.[24]

To the extent that real political power is implicated in post-apartheid AIDS conspiracy stories, it appears to be supranational, i.e., located in sources of power beyond and greater than that of the new South African government—notably the United States and its associated (pharmaceutical) corporate interests. That South African citizens and their government are perceived as subject to powerful international forces probably reflects broader anxieties about international economic integration and the concomitant restrictions on domestic policy. The ANC had, soon after the process of constitutional negotiations began in the early 1990s, largely abandoned its revolutionary rhetoric about nationalization and "disciplining" capital in favor of more open economic and business-friendly policies.[25] Rather than speaking of growth through redistribution, the new government soon stressed the dangers of capital flight and the need to combat poverty through growth. The post-apartheid political context was thus one of constrained optimism about what the state could achieve, in addition to increasing alarm about the rapid growth of HIV infections and AIDS deaths. It was, in short, a cultural context probably ripe for the spread of stories about powerful, probably US-based, scientists spreading harm. The idea that HIV may have been manufactured specifically as a US bioweapon thus may have seemed plausible to many and could have entered the popular culture without much ecotypical modification.

The post-apartheid context was also one in which the power of science was being felt in more intimate ways, not only with regard to the HIV epidemic, with its complicated testing and treatment regimens, but also in the genetic engineering of food. This may also have generated new insecurities, perhaps with ramifications for how people think about the origin of HIV. For example, in a focus group discussion among AIDS conspiracy believers in Cape Town,[26] one of them explained:

> I think it comes from scientists. It seems it was created in a lab. Because even a lot of food when it is planted, they put chemicals in it so that it grows

in different ways. So when you mix chemicals and then mix people with that, and cows also eat that same mixture and meat, the entire eco-system is changed. . . . So that is why there are diseases we do not know origins of—that just come out of nowhere. . . .

Sometimes I can read something new and have my doubts, but most of the time my main view is that people who made it and research on worldly things are the scientists. Because they can still research a cure. And they are still inventing new things for people to live better, but they still don't know how it will change and do what. (Focus Group Participant Number 3)

These comments suggest a distinct ambiguity toward science in that it is both distrusted (for meddling with nature) and recognized to be powerful, perhaps even to the point of developing a cure for HIV. But even so, the process of scientific experimentation is clearly perceived as fraught with danger. A fellow focus group participant agreed, also pointing to scientific experimentation as a source of suspicion for the origins of HIV:

So what they did—I'm not saying, no one knows, we are all still searching as to where it came from—it's just my view that it came from scientists. So they did whatever remedy they made and they tested it on people— whichever people they tested it on and then it gave them this disease of AIDS. So what I'm saying is that it was tested on humans and then this AIDS happened. (Focus Group Participant Number 4)

In his detailed exploration of a black South African man's suspicions about HIV testing and treatment, Jonny Steinberg observes that his subject's strongest suspicion was that HIV originated in the "vividly imagined laboratories of Western science." But Steinberg also emphasizes that he was "entirely open" to other possibilities, to gathering new evidence and wondering what one should be looking out for.[27] A similar openness and ambivalence was evident in the Cape Town focus group. Despite having indicated on the survey questionnaire that they "strongly agreed" with AIDS conspiracy theories, the subsequent discussion reveals a much more fluid set of attitudes. Participants were more concerned with the gaps in our scientific knowledge, the potential for experiments to go awry, and the confusing aspects of HIV's pathogenesis than they were about AIDS origin conspiracy theories.

Paul Farmer, a physician and medical anthropologist who wrote a seminal book on AIDS stigma and the Haitian experience, argues that AIDS conspiracy theories are the counter-theories to stigma and blame for the epidemic and are best understood as "symbolic rejoinders of the scapegoats."[28] Interestingly, this dynamic was not evident in the Cape Town focus group. The participants accepted as self-evident that sexual behavior was the main problem. They blamed poverty and the "stress" of having to put food on the table for "lack of thinking" and "carelessness" among their fellow black South Africans when it came to safe sexual behavior. The closest any of them got to suggesting that HIV may have been deliberately introduced to harm black people was to wonder whether the scientists had done "studies" of African sexual behavior and therefore knew that it would spread particularly quickly among them.

But in raising questions and testing theories on each other, the role of political leadership came to the fore as an important issue in the discussion. Respondents argued that whatever doubts one might have about the veracity of some official messages about HIV prevention and treatment, most people had little option other than to trust what they were being told by political leaders. As discussed in more detail in chapter 5, this was particularly problematic in South Africa, where both President Mbeki and his health minister Tshabalala-Msimang promoted AIDS conspiracy narratives while delaying the use of antiretrovirals in the public sector. While neither came close to what Richard Hofstadter famously called the "paranoid style" of politics,[29] they were deeply suspicious of HIV science. Hofstadter wrote that "the distinguishing thing about the paranoid style is not that its exponents see conspiracies or plots here or there in history, but that they regard a 'vast' or 'gigantic' conspiracy *as the motive force* in historical events."[30] Mbeki and Tshabalala-Msimang rather saw AIDS as one of those "plots here and there in history."

Mbeki actively evoked AIDS conspiracy theories by alleging that the CIA, working with the large pharmaceutical companies, was part of a conspiracy seeking to promote the view that HIV was the sole cause of

AIDS and that toxic antiretrovirals were the only treatment.[31] Even though Mbeki later withdrew from public discussion on AIDS in the face of resistance from within the ANC and from civil society, notably the Treatment Action Campaign (TAC), his supporters continued to promote suspicion about the origins of HIV, some hinting that it was the product of deliberate biowarfare. As late as 2006, the political executive in charge of health in the KwaZulu-Natal Province, Peggy Nkonyeni, drew connections between "this thing called bioterrorism or biological warfare" and HIV.[32]

Tshabalala-Msimang, however, drew on other conspiracy theorists whose paranoid style was much more global and in line with what Hofstadter had in mind. Most notably, she sparked controversy in 2000 by circulating extracts from *Behold a Pale Horse* by the American conspiracy theorist William Cooper.[33] In so doing, she illustrated how ideas from the broader international "cultic milieu" can cross political, cultural, and national boundaries.

FUSION PARANOIA: ECLECTIC IDEOLOGICAL BORROWINGS ACROSS THE ATLANTIC

Cooper believed that AIDS is part of a gigantic historical conspiracy involving the US government working in cahoots with aliens from outer space, Jews, Freemasons, and the Illuminati (an imaginary ancient secret society of elites).[34] He was, in the words of Michael Barkun, a "bridging" theorist, who was able to speak both to Ufologists and antigovernment militants,[35] thereby attracting new audiences for his conspiracy theories. According to Cooper, HIV was created by the US military and the CIA and injected into the African population during the 1970s through a smallpox eradication campaign, and into the African-American and homosexual population through hepatitis-B vaccinations. He argued that this was part of a Club of Rome plot to address global overpopulation and that "the elite" had been provided with a prophylaxis. He also asserted that a cure for AIDS existed, but would only be released when enough people had died. Already influential for being "much read in both UFO and militia circles,"[36] *Behold a*

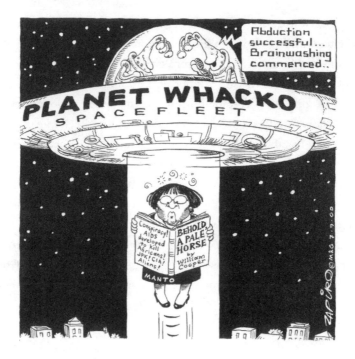

FIGURE 2.3 Critical media coverage of Manto Tshabalala-Msimang's promotion of William Cooper's book (cartoon by Zapiro, Sept. 8, 2000, in the *Mail and Guardian*, Johannesburg). © Zapiro. Reprinted with permission.

Pale Horse was, through Tshabalala-Msimang, now provided an influential airing in the highest reaches of the South African government—and was widely discussed in the media and on the radio (fig. 2.3).

As is evident from his writings and broadcasts,[37] Cooper was a right-wing misogynist libertarian who believed that people had been turned into "cattle" by governments and that only the truly enlightened, who could see the interplanetary conspiracy for what it was and were prepared to resist the state in all forms, could genuinely be free. His paranoia ranged from the global to the personal in that he believed he was being targeted by "The Illuminati Socialist President of the United States of America, William Jefferson Clinton" as well as "by the bogus and unconstitutional Internal Revenue Service."[38] Living a life true to his views, Cooper was eventually indicted on federal charges after refusing to pay taxes and then declared a "major fugitive" by the US Marshals Service when he failed to appear in court. Local law enforcement officials dragged their heels in executing the warrant, but after he threatened a fellow citizen with a weapon, sheriffs tried to arrest him. Cooper resisted, shot the law enforcement officer, and was killed in the ensuring gunfight.[39] His supporters believe he was assassinated by the very conspiracy he was exposing.[40]

This link between Tshabalala-Msimang and Cooper illustrates how the creation and propagation of AIDS origin conspiracy theories can entail connections, if only in the sphere of ideas, between those with very different views of the world and their place in it. That a government official in a middle-income country committed to using the power of the state to facilitate income redistribution was promoting the ideas of an antistate US militia leader and acknowledged source of inspiration for the US terrorist Timothy McVeigh[41]—and who was preparing US "patriots" for an alien invasion—is strange indeed. That she had dedicated her life to the anti-apartheid movement, whereas he reportedly supported the Ku Klux Klan,[42] makes it all the more so.

Yet there are other such politically incongruous connections in the world of AIDS conspiracy theory. For example, the white right-winger and AIDS conspiracy theorist Leonard Horowitz[43] has links with Louis Farrakhan,[44] the leader of the Nation of Islam (chapter 3), and is an acknowledged influence on Jeremiah Wright (Barack Obama's pastor, who claimed that HIV is a US-manufactured bioweapon).[45] Horowitz promotes a range of medical conspiracy theories, including about the laboratory origin of HIV, in books, videos, and on his own television station.[46] This serves to cast doubt on scientific medicine—thereby conveniently boosting the demand for the "alternative" healing products he sells over the Internet.[47] In this regard, Horowitz is a classic example of the cultropreneurs who promote and benefit from conspiracy theories about HIV science (chapter 6). Conspiracy theory features prominently in the promotion of "Oxysilver"[48] (a mineral water retailing at the discount price of $533.52 for 144 ounces), which supposedly supports the immune system by transmitting healing "vibrations" to the body and whose "healing ability is obviously demonstrated by the greenish-yellow color of most of the botanical world."[49] Having initially claimed that it actually destroyed "disease forming bacteria, viruses and fungi in your body," Horowitz was forced to amend his website after the Food and Drug Administration (FDA) acted on complaints about it.[50] The advertising now reads that Oxysilver "could actually free the world from BigPharma's deadliest manipulations, medical intoxications and petro-chemical environmental pollutions" and that it "destroys [FDA Censored Word] and common chronic [FDA Censored Word] largely attributable to weakened immune systems."

Some commentators suggest that shared attitudes, such as anti-Semi-tism or racial separatism, account for the seemingly incongruous connec-tions between white right-wingers such as Cooper and Horowitz, and black nationalists like Tshabalala-Msimang and Farrakhan.[51] Others, such as sociologist Colin Campbell,[52] argue that ideologically strange bedfellows are characteristic of what he termed the broader "cultic milieu" in which countercultural practitioners, be they spiritualists, alternative healers, con-spiracy theorists, or militia members, are united in a common opposition to the dominant culture.[53]

The idea that conspiracy theory transcends political boundaries actu-ally originates with Hofstadter, who noted that the paranoid style was also evident in right-wing and fascist movements as well as in Stalinist Russia and the left-wing press.[54] Various other commentators in the broader con-spiracy theory literature have also noted how many conspiracy theories find support across the social and political spectrum. Journalist Michael Kelly refers to this phenomenon as "fusion paranoia" in which the left/right dis-tinction is replaced with the more primitive "Us" (the people) versus "Them" (the people who control the people) polarity: "From this fundamental as-sumption, fusion paranoia builds to an array of related beliefs: that the gov-erning elite lies as a matter of course; that it is controlled by people acting in concert against the common good and at the bidding of powerful interests working behind the scenes and that it routinely commits acts of appalling treachery."[55] Specifically with regard to beliefs such as AIDS being a gov-ernment plot to kill off black people and homosexuals, Kelly observes that "there is no left and no right here, only unanimity of belief in the boundless cabalistic evil of the government and its allies."[56]

In constructing narratives about the nature of that boundless cabalistic evil, conspiracy theorists often borrow from each other. As policy analyst

Chip Bertlet puts it, "Conspiracy theories are not merely additive mélanges: they are less like a conspiracist Pot-au-feu and more like a meal selected from a smörgåsbord of conspiratorial snacks."[57] In terms of this approach, there is no necessary contradiction between Tshabala-Msimang selecting aspects of Cooper's grand conspiratorial narrative to shed doubt on the mainstream scientific account of the origins of HIV. She was, in this account, merely dabbling in the cultic milieu and 'snacking' at the table of conspiracy theory.

ORIGINS OF THE IDEA THAT HIV IS A US BIOWEAPON: SOVIET MISINFORMATION

By the time that President Mbeki voiced his suspicions in 2000 about the role of the CIA in promoting misinformation about HIV, the idea of HIV as a US/CIA-manufactured bioweapon had been recorded in Europe, the United States, Africa, and the Caribbean.[58] Ironically, this conspiratorial ecotype can be traced to a *real* conspiracy, notably a deliberate and coordinated East German and Soviet Union misinformation campaign.

As far back as 1987, the US State Department claimed that the Soviet Union was behind the "HIV as US bioweapon" story.[59] But it was only after a KGB officer admitted the Soviet role in spreading AIDS conspiracy theories and two former Stasi officers published a book in 1992 describing how they had "collaborated with the KGB to spin the AIDS yarn, using [Russian-born biophysicist Jakob] Segal and his scientific credentials to lend the story credence"[60] that the existence of the misinformation campaign was corroborated by inside sources. In the meantime, the story circulated around the world, sometimes with the proviso that it had been "accused" of being a Soviet misinformation plot.

The disinformation campaign appears to have started in 1983 (i.e., even before it was proven that any virus caused AIDS) with the publication of a letter in a pro-Soviet New Delhi newspaper, *The Patriot*, accusing the US army of manufacturing the AIDS virus in its bacteriological laboratory in Fort Detrick, Maryland (an old National Guard airfield about an hour's drive from Washington, D.C.).[61] The story was given further impetus in 1985 when the Russian *Literaturnaya Gazeta* repeated and refined the allegations, bolstering them with a report by Jakob Segal, then retired from East Berlin's Humboldt University, and his wife Lilli. They claimed that US scientists based at Fort Detrick had, in 1977, used genetic technology to splice and combine the leukemia virus Visna, found in sheep, with the human leukemia virus HTLV-1 to create a new infectious AIDS-causing pathogen. The new virus supposedly entered the general population after being tested on prisoners.[62]

An extended version of the Segals' claims was circulated in Zimbabwe in 1986 at the time of the Non-aligned Movement summit in Harare, sparking sympathetic reviews in newspapers in Zimbabwe, Kenya, and Senegal.[63] The story reached its apex in the first six months of 1987, when it made the front page of the London *Sunday Express*, was broadcast by Dan Rather on the CBS evening news, and disseminated throughout the world.[64] William Campbell Douglass was the first to pick up on the story and transform it for US audiences. His particular spin, that HIV was a communist-controlled US-manufactured bioweapon, proved particularly popular in the African-American community[65]—which is why David Gilbert concentrated on it in his subsequent debunking of AIDS conspiracy theory (chapter 4).

The United States responded to the disinformation by complaining to the Soviet Union and publishing in July 1987 an exposé of the campaign and a scientific rebuttal including commentary from Luc Montagnier, the codiscoverer of HIV.[66] According to Russian sources, the following month President Mikhail Gorbachev instructed the KGB to desist, and the Soviet news agency stopped reporting the story.[67] But by that time the story had gained an independent life of its own, spawning the many varieties and ecotypes that persist today.

SCIENCE, VACCINES, AND THE ORIGINS OF HIV

One of the reasons for the "HIV as US bioweapon" theory's international traction was the uncertainty at the time about the true origins of HIV. As

Christopher Hitchens has astutely observed, conspiracy theory is the "white noise which moves in to fill the vacuity of the official version" and that "to blame the theorist is therefore to look at only half the story, and sometimes even less."[68] And in this respect, there have been gaps and uncertainties in the scientific explanation of the origin of HIV, uncertainties that are only recently being addressed through evolutionary genetic research.

Early speculation that HIV originated in Africa from contact with monkeys had, by the late 1980s, resulted in highly racialized (if not racist) media coverage,[69] thus creating the context for the bioweapon narrative to flourish as a rejoinder. And, in the 1990s, when suspicions were aroused that HIV may have entered the African population through a contaminated polio vaccine, this probably reinforced, for many people, their skepticism and doubt about the emerging "official" scientific explanation—that HIV evolved after SIV jumped the species barrier through the hunting of primates as bushmeat, the so-called "cut hunter" theory.

The polio-vaccine theory of the origin of AIDS emerged in the early 1990s in a series of magazine articles and letters to journals[70] suggesting that SIV may have entered the human population through a polio-vaccine trial conducted in the Congo in the late 1950s. But it was only when journalist Edward Hooper investigated the story, and linked the first known samples of HIV infection to areas where the vaccine trial had been conducted in a detailed book called *The River: A Journey to the Source of HIV and AIDS*,[71] that the theory gained greater coverage and popular credence.

Given that vaccinations have in the past been associated with disease transmission (for example, faulty vaccinations have transmitted schistosomiasis, hepatitis B, and even polio),[72] the idea of such an iatrogenic (physician-caused) disease was not unreasonable. Furthermore, by suggesting that the African HIV epidemic was the unintended consequence of a vaccination campaign, it was not a conspiracy theory in the strong sense of the term. To the extent that a conspiratorial move is made, it is to assert that the truth about HIV's accidental origins is being covered up by the scientific community today.

According to Hooper, HIV arose from the use of chimpanzee cells to grow the experimental polio vaccine. Given the known link between a strain of SIV (SIVcp2) and one strain of HIV (HIV-1) as well as the practice of using primate cells to grow vaccine cultures, the polio-vaccine theory of HIV-1's origin was plausible. Hooper's suspicion was that the vaccine trial used chimpanzee cells as a vaccine substrate, thereby facilitating the cross-species transmission of SIVcp2 to HIV-1. As SIV-infected chimpanzees had, by this stage, been found to be the source of HIV-1, the scientific community took the claims seriously, and several independent investigations into the remaining vaccine samples were conducted.

This culminated in a contentious meeting hosted by the Royal Society, at which scientists concluded (over Hooper's protests) that his theory was unlikely to be correct because none of the remaining samples tested positive for human or simian viruses, none of the scientists involved in the trial could recall chimpanzee cells being used in vaccine production, and because emerging research on the genetic evolution of HIV suggested that the transmission to humans occurred long before the late 1950s when the vaccine trial had been conducted.[73] Hooper responded by saying that none of the tested vaccine samples had actually been produced in Africa (hence the tests were irrelevant—even though he had earlier called for them) and that he had new "smoking guns," namely recollections by some of the Africans involved in the project that chimpanzee cells had been used. Stanley Plotkin, who had helped test the vaccine, responded by saying that he had contacted former colleagues who had testified in writing that they had never worked with chimpanzee cells. He concluded: "There is no gun. There is no bullet. There is no shooter. There is no motive. There is only smoke created by Mr. Hooper."[74] Hooper, however, suspected a cover-up. He told science journalist Jon Cohen that he would not give up "until I am certain that Science is really going to investigate the issue properly, fully and honestly." Cohen, however, concluded that his "dire portrait of capital-S science" was overdrawn and unwarranted: "A group of devoted scientists, albeit a small one, has been addressing the issue properly, fully and honestly. That Hooper finds their work wanting reveals more about him than about the scientists and their efforts."[75]

Hooper continues to promote his theory on websites and through further elaborations about the "evidence" and what he portrays as the reprehensible tactics of scientists to avoid it.[76] He believes he has been accorded insufficient respect by the scientific establishment, and some social scientists agree.[77] But although the polio-vaccine theory cannot be conclusively disproved, keeping it alive involves ever more convoluted hypotheses. For example, phylogeographic analysis pinpoints the probable source of the viruses that gave rise to the HIV-1 group M epidemic (responsible for over 90 percent of HIV infections worldwide) as being chimpanzees in the extreme southeast corner of Cameroon.[78] One thus has to assume that hunters responded to the supposed demand for chimpanzees from the vaccine trial in the Congo by hunting them in the Cameroon and shipping them downriver to the Congo. Furthermore, one has to confront the challenge of finding a separate set of vaccine incidents to account for the separate zoonotic transmission of HIV-2 from sooty mangabey monkeys to humans, a most difficult task given that scientists now believe that HIV-2 entered humans through at least eight separate transmissions.[79] And one also has to reject all the evolutionary biological studies that date the origin of HIV-1 before the 1950s.

By studying the genetic diversity of HIV, scientists have been able to conduct a "molecular clock" analysis, which dates the most recent common ancestor of HIV-1 group M to between 1908 and 1941.[80] This entails computer modeling of the rate of evolution of the virus, but what makes it particularly compelling is that the predictions of the models match the genetic characteristics of viral samples dating from 1959 and 1960 in the Congo (Democratic Republic of the Congo, or the DRC). It now seems most likely that SIV has been crossing into the human population for a long time, but that it was the rapid urbanization of the post–World War II period which turned previously isolated episodes into a burgeoning epidemic.[81] Other plausible supplementary transmission mechanisms include iatrogenic factors, notably the reuse of hypodermic needles and arm-to-arm vaccinations in the early colonial period.[82]

Whatever the balance between biological, social, and iatrogenic factors, we do know that HIV-1 originated in Africa long before scientists in Fort Detrick supposedly manufactured it in the mid-1970s, and well before science had developed anywhere near the capacity to genetically engineer one. But the important issue here is not whether the "AIDS as genocidal bioweapon" claims are wrong (which they are), but rather why they were, and remain, thinkable for many people.

WHY IS IT THINKABLE THAT THE UNITED STATES
MANUFACTURED HIV AS A BIOWEAPON?

Despite its origins in a Soviet–East German misinformation campaign, the "HIV as US bioweapon" theory disseminated around the world in part because it sounded plausible. The United States had indeed operated a biological weapons program at Fort Detrick, which had produced anthrax bombs in 1944 and a range of germ warfare weapons that had only narrowly avoided being used in World War II.[83] This research continued after the war, and by 1960 Fort Detrick had become the largest consumer of guinea pigs in the world.[84] The army also tested their biological weapon delivery systems on unsuspecting human populations. For example, in the 1950s Fort Detrick developed the capacity to produce millions of mosquitoes and infect them with yellow fever. To test whether mosquitoes could be fired out of a warhead and then go on to bite people, the army carried out tests involving the release of uninfected mosquitoes over Savannah (Georgia) and then in Florida.[85] Between 1948 and 1968, two hundred secret experiments involving dummy germ warfare attacks were conducted, including in 1966 on New York City using harmless bacteria.[86]

In 1971, President Richard Nixon ordered that the offensive biological weapons program be discontinued and all stockpiles of harmful substances destroyed. However some biowarfare research continued in the guise of developing supposedly "defensive" rather than "offensive" weapons.[87] For most of the 1970s, the facility at Fort Detrick focused on cancer research, with many of the researchers previously engaged in bioweapons development joining mainstream scientists to explore potential viral causes of cancer. Despite being a civilian program, it had obvious military applications. Potential cancer-causing viruses were collected, grown, and tested on animals, and the aerosol distribution of carcinogenic viruses was studied.[88] Particularly relevant for AIDS conspiracy theories is the fact that Robert Gallo, who subsequently codiscovered HIV and developed a test for it, was a project officer for the viral cancer program in which monkeys were infected with viruses, human cancer tissues, and even sheep's blood in an effort to find transmissible cancers.[89] The Soviet misinformation story thus harnessed a grain of truth (Gallo was indeed funded by the program, and sheep's blood was reportedly used by some researchers, though not Gallo) to add a patina of plausibility to the implausible claim that HIV was created by scientists.

The Gallo link was subsequently picked up and embellished by Horowitz and woven into his evolving conspiratorial account of the origin of AIDS. In a video (available on YouTube)[90] labeled: "Robert Gallo: The Man That [sic] Created AIDS," Horowitz includes a confrontation between himself and Gallo at the 1996 Vancouver International AIDS conference. It records Horowitz suggesting to Gallo that his experiments may have given "rise to the AIDS virus" by contaminating monkeys with a new pathogen he supposedly engineered from the human leukemia virus and chicken sarcoma and other animal viruses. In Horowitz's wide-eyed conspiratorial account, this new virus was injected into monkeys subsequently used to produce a hepatitis B vaccine, which spread HIV to humans. He accompanies his video production with camera shots of two of Gallo's papers supposedly "proving" he did this (they do nothing of the kind)[91] and asserting that Gallo had used a monkey virus (SV40—which causes cancer in hamsters but not people) to facilitate the process. Gallo gapes in astonishment, then erupts in frustration, telling Horowitz his claims are "beyond asinine" and that his theory was all "pineapples, kiwis, grapes and cherries, mixed in with some other tooty-fruity." Horowitz continues, undeterred, until Gallo interrupts him, sarcastically saying: "Yes, we did. Everything was created by us, working in a laboratory." But he then goes on more seriously, pointing out that

> No scientist could have deliberately created it unless he was a super genius and ten years ahead of his time. The AIDS virus definitively existed long before molecular cloning. That is point one. Point two, we know the full sequence. The genome of HIV was published by our lab in 1985 and in Paris at the same time. The genome has no homology to any known existing virus in the world except SIV discovered after it. It has nothing to do with cats, with chicken sarcoma virus. SV40 is a DNA virus that comes from little animals that can transform cells in culture. It has no sequences in HIV. Further, we have never worked with SV40 with those viruses together, and

if we did, the whole thing would be irrelevant. I think you need to begin
with biology 101 high school.

Horowitz, however, has the words "unproven defense," "lie," and "he did"
floating across the screen as Gallo talks.

Aside from targeting the man who developed the first HIV test and
codiscovered HIV, the KGB-Stasi misinformation was brilliant also for
another grain of truth it harnessed—notably the US military's expressed
desire to create novel pathogens. Dr. Donald MacArthur, the deputy director of the Department of Defense, had testified in 1969 before a House
of Representatives subcommittee on military appropriations about the
army's interest in "developing a new infective micro-organism." Horowitz, unsurprisingly, highlights this testimony in his video before linking
Gallo to the story as the agent who was employed to develop the new
organism.

Note that the idea of creating a new infective micro-organism is not
particularly far-fetched. As Robert Harris and Jeremy Paxman observe,
MacArthur's desire was "not merely academic speculation" because that
year the British Army Biological Warfare Laboratory at Porton Down had
collaborated with Fort Detrick to transfer (successfully) genes between different strains of the plague bacillus.[92] In his testimony MacArthur reported
that the army believed it would have been possible to create a new infectious
organism for $10 million within five to ten years, but that the project had
not been taken forward because of funding constraints and a reluctance to
involve outside researchers in "such a controversial endeavor."[93] Still, to the
suspiciously minded, the MacArthur testimony was the smoking gun that
proved the laboratory origin of AIDS. In the words of Boyd "Ed" Graves,
the now deceased HIV-positive African-American who tried to sue the US
government for manufacturing HIV, MacArthur's testimony was "direct
credible evidence" that the United States had "engineered AIDS."[94] This,
coupled with his suspicions about the special viral cancer program at Fort
Detrick (discussed below), led him to conclude that "we have found the
origin of AIDS, it is our nation state, it is us."[95]

The mere fact that the United States ran a biological weapons program
which may have included research on cancer-causing viruses was probably

not sufficient on its own to generate the high public levels of endorsement of AIDS origin beliefs reported in table 2.1. The publicity generated in the mid-1970s by investigations into abuses by the Federal Bureau of Investigation (FBI) and the CIA (the House Select Committee on Intelligence, aka the "Pike Committee" and the Senate's "Church Committee") was crucial in creating a climate of suspicion toward secret government scientific testing programs. During the hearings of the Church Committee (named after its chairman, Frank Church) it was revealed that there were CIA assassination plots against foreign leaders which were either unsuccessful (against Castro in Cuba) or successfully carried out by dissidents supported by the CIA (Lumumba in Zaire and Trujillo in the Dominican Republic) and that the CIA had developed the capacity to disable people with drugs, chemicals, and biological agents.[96] The committee also found that the CIA had, in clear contravention of Nixon's orders, stockpiled a cache of deadly biological weapons in a vault codenamed MK-Naomi containing substances such as shellfish toxin, anthrax, encephalitis and cobra venom in sufficient quantities to "destroy the population of a small city."[97] As George Marcus points out in the introduction to his volume *Paranoia within Reason*, these sorts of covert activities related to the Cold War against communism reflected genuinely "paranoid policies of statecraft and governing habits of thought" which rendered it "quite reasonable and commonsensical" for people to adopt conspiracy theories toward government involvement with the public.[98]

Frank Church played to the media, likening the CIA to a "rogue elephant on the rampage."[99] He provided reporters with a highly publicized photo-opportunity when releasing details of a biological weapon delivery system supposedly accurate up to 250 feet (fig. 2.4). This "ultimate murder weapon, able to kill without sound and with barely a trace" involved applying poison to a tiny dart the size of a sewing needle ("a non-discernable micro-bio-inoculater"), then using an electric dart gun (a "noise free disseminator" resembling a large .45 pistol with an electronic sight) to propel the dart silently toward the victim.[100]

That these revelations echoed through popular culture and shaped AIDS conspiracy accounts is easy to see. Cooper located the origin of AIDS firmly within MK-Naomi, but Graves took the matter more personally.

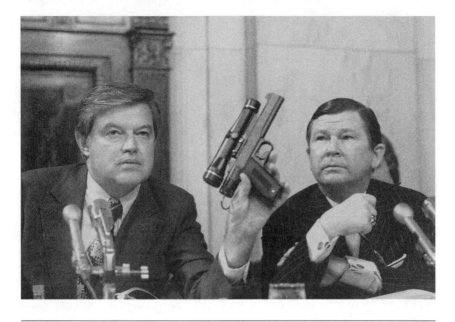

FIGURE 2.4 Senator Frank Church (*left*) and Senator John Tower and poison dart gun at 1975 Senate Committee hearing. (*Photo:* Henry Griffin, Associated Press)

African-American journalist LeRoy Whitfield, who interviewed Graves for a long piece he wrote on AIDS conspiracy theories, reports that Graves accepted the possibility of having been infected with HIV through sex but

> more likely, he believes, he was the victim of a stealth dart gun, a "micro-bio-inoculater" that can tag unsuspecting victims from 100 feet away without so much as a prick, a product of the U.S. government's biological warfare program. Or, he imagines, he may have been one of thousands of unlucky African Americans infected through a bite by a virus-distributing mosquito bred by government contractors at an island facility off the shores of Manhattan. Or: "The HIV virus is the result of a century-long hunt for a contagious cancer that selectively kills." "If they didn't want me to discover the true origins of AIDS," Graves says, cutting a glare in my direction, "they shouldn't have given it to me."[101]

Graves's particular ecotype of the AIDS origin conspiracy theory clearly borrows from the Senate hearings and the Soviet–East German misinformation story, as well as various accounts—notably Horowitz's—of how HIV entered the US African-American and homosexual populations through vaccine programs.[102] Graves explicitly acknowledges a debt to Horowitz[103] for pointing him toward the cancer virus program at Fort Detrick. Other sources appear to be William Campbell Douglass as well as Alan Cantwell (a dermatologist from Los Angeles who claims that HIV was deliberately injected into the black and homosexual population during hepatitis B vaccine trials in New York in the late 1970s).[104]

Following Douglass's and Horowitz's lead, Graves implicates Gallo by claiming that he helped develop HIV in Fort Detrick and accusing Gallo also of assisting the US government to inoculate monkeys with HIV and releasing them into the wild.[105] And, borrowing from Cooper, Graves claimed that a cure for AIDS existed, but was being kept secret by the government. In coming to this conclusion, Graves relied heavily the "research logic" spelled out in a flow chart in Report 8 of the government-sponsored Special Cancer Virus Program, stating that if a new viral pathogen was discovered, work could only continue on it once a cure was available. The chart outlined various "phases" from the selection of specimens, to establishing their replication, disease causation, and immunological response, and finally to phase 4, which required that the research only proceed if "control of disease and/or virus replication in animals and/or tissue culture has been demonstrated." For Graves, the very existence of this flow chart (which he presented on his website[106] and to various audiences) proved the laboratory origin of AIDS and that a secret cure existed.[107] But all it actually proves is that a research protocol had been drawn up to prevent scientists from proceeding with the development of a potential bioweapon unless a cure was available.

Graves produced a book detailing his conspiracy theory,[108] spoke at community events, and operated a website promoting these views. He also reportedly engaged "independent filmmaker" Brent Leung (discussed also in chapter 6) to make a documentary on his discovery,[109] though it is unclear if this was ever made. He petitioned his congressional representatives to get the government to investigate the Special Cancer Virus Program,[110]

and he launched several unsuccessful legal actions against the US government to identify the origins of HIV and the cure he believed was being kept
secret. His lawsuits, however, were thrown out of court as being factually
inaccurate and without foundation.

Later, Graves came to believe that Gallo had given the AIDS cure[111] to
Marvin Antelman, a conspiracy theorist who believes that the Illuminati,
Jewish traitors, and communists are involved in a global plot to oppress
Jews and Christians.[112] Antelman supposedly patented this cure under the
name Tetrasil (later, Imusil), along with a range of alternative by-products
all based on the same claim: that tetrasilver tetroxide (Ag_4O_4), a disinfec-
tant used in swimming pools, will kill a range of pathogens.[113] (Strangely
enough, these are similar claims to those made by Horowitz for Oxysilver.)
Preliminary tests of Tetrasil were apparently conducted in Honduras on a
few patients (some of whom developed liver problems) and possibly also in
South Africa where they were reportedly monitored by a "top S. African
Executive."[114] Gerald Pierone, a doctor who responds to questions on www
.thebody.com, reviewed the patent reports, saying that they were "beyond
imagination," that the trials were inadequate and unethical, and that given
the reported side effects (especially hepatomegaly, or enlargement of the
liver), people should "stay away from this stuff like the plague!"[115]

Graves, however, believed in the cure to the point of volunteering himself for this experimental treatment and subsequently promoted it in Zambia and other African countries.[116] In 2004 he told an interviewer from the
Nation of Islam's publication *Final Call*:

> There is a tetra silver that is used in swimming pools. We found a similarity
> of the blood in your body with respect to the water in a swimming pool.
> If you put something in a disc in your swimming pool, then all the water
> becomes clear. The same is true with this one-time injection of purifying the
> blood in the body. The process is identical to how you purify the water in
> the swimming pool, and I believe that the swimming pool product is called
> tetra silver. Dr Antelman changed the name from Tetrasil to Imusil.[117]

Despite believing strongly in this cure, Graves died after a long illness (presumably AIDS) in 2009 at age 57.

Graves was named one of the twenty-five most influential people in Cleveland by *Cleveland Life*, Ohio's largest African-American newspaper, in March 1999 and was certainly not alone in promoting AIDS conspiracy theories. More prominent African-Americans have promoted or validated AIDS conspiracy theories on the airways and in the media. These include Louis Farrakhan and Jeremiah Wright (as mentioned earlier) as well as film and media stars such as Will Smith, Spike Lee, Bill Cosby, and Tony Brown.[118] This leads us to the obvious next question: why is the idea thinkable that the US government conspired to create HIV to harm black people in particular?

THE HISTORICAL CONTEXT OF RACIALIZED SUSPICION

The history of racial discrimination and oppression of black people in the United States, notably slavery and Jim Crow laws, is an obvious context for the persistent belief that the US government conspires with powerful collaborators to harm African-Americans.[119] Certainly the revelations during the House and Senate Committee hearings during the mid-1970s would have done little to dampen any such suspicions. The public heard that the FBI had carried out investigations into hundreds of thousands of "subversives" (many of them black) between 1960 and 1974, had incited murder and other violence among African-Americans through the use of anonymous FBI letters, had infiltrated black organizations, and harassed families of activists—all as part of a government program known as COINTELPRO ("counter-intelligence program").

COINTELPRO was directed at political radicals in the United States, notably the Black Panther Party, but also toward such leftist groups as the Socialist Workers Party and civil rights campaigners like Martin Luther King.[120] It seems to have entailed surveillance, infiltration, petty arrests, and spreading false rumors (to disrupt relations within black organizations and between them and their white allies).[121] What the Pike Committee referred to as "FBI racism," other commentators have concluded was much more sinister than that, raising questions about the possible involvement of the FBI in King's death and calling for an independent investigation into the case.[122]

Even mainstream observers were shocked by the revelations about COINTELPRO. In his memoirs of his time serving on the Church Committee, Loch Johnson wrote:

> I thought of the boast sent to bureau headquarters by an FBI office in southern California during the 1960s: "Shootings, beatings and a high degree of unrest continues to prevail in the ghetto area of southeast San Diego," read the memo. "Although no specific counterintelligence action can be credited with contributing to this overall situation, it is felt that a substantial amount of the unrest is directly attributable to the [COINTELPRO] program." If the philosophy behind such extreme use of secret government power were acceptable, then it seemed every conceivable intrusion into the rights of private citizens could be anticipated.[123]

Other secret CIA programs, known as MK-Delta and MK-Ultra, were exposed through legal action in the early 1970s and through the Senate and House investigations in 1975. The public heard that scientists and anthropologists had been used unwittingly by the CIA as part of a broader thrust to develop techniques of mind control and torture, some of which found their way into the CIA's interrogation manual.[124] The public also heard how an MK-Ultra project, established in 1953 for the covert use of biological and chemical weapons, tested a large number of drugs on drug addicts seeking care in a Kentucky clinic. Most of the patients were "negro males" and most of the experiments involved the unwitting receipt of LSD.[125] This would have resonated in the black community in particular, given the revelations that surfaced in the mid-1970s about the now infamous Tuskegee Study, which left black syphilis patients in rural Alabama deliberately untreated for three decades (1932–1972) in order to study the natural progression of the disease.[126] As Harlon Dalton observes—explicitly with regard to conspiracy beliefs about AIDS—the history of slavery, discrimination, and medical abuse such as Tuskegee rendered "no depredation on the part of the government unthinkable."[127]

Two decades after the Pike and Church Committee investigations into the CIA and FBI, a new scare about the CIA and its evil intent toward the black community was generated by the publication in August 1996 of a three-part series by Gary Webb in the *San Jose Mercury News* drawing a link between the CIA and drug gangs in San Francisco and Los Angeles.[128] Entitled "Dark Alliance," Webb's articles claimed that the CIA knew about drug dealing by Nicaraguan contras in Los Angeles ("the CIA's army"), but did not stop them because it was an important source of funding for them. This, he suggested, resulted in a crack cocaine explosion in urban America, which in turn enabled the gangs to buy weapons. Further investigation by the *Washington Post*, the *Los Angeles Times*, and the *New York Times* (and by a CIA review and a Senate Intelligence Committee) found no evidence for the claim, and the *Mercury News* later backtracked, removing the CIA insignia from its website and stating that it only meant that individuals associated with the CIA were selling crack.[129]

Daniel Hellinger observes that this story resonated with the African-American community in part because the "facts seemed to fit the theory." He notes that there are documented cases of the CIA's involvement in the drug trade,[130] and argues that Webb's story drew ire because it challenged the notion that these were aberrant (rather than regular) CIA activities. In any event, the story created sufficient concern that African-American politicians and the CIA leadership felt it necessary to hold town meetings in several urban centers. That the story had fueled related suspicions about the government's dirty dealings against African-Americans in general is evident from a Los Angeles town meeting convened by Rep. Maxine Waters (D-CA). Whitfield reports that at the meeting a woman said: "Black men are in jail for selling drugs the CIA brought to our community the same way they brought the guns here for us to kill each other. If they don't get you that way, government doctors will stick you with AIDS. One way or another, they will destroy us."[131]

But while AIDS conspiracy beliefs are thinkable for a range of historical reasons, it is important to bear in mind that they remain minority viewpoints even in populations where levels of endorsement appear to be relatively high. Furthermore, it is often very difficult to trace an exact path from specific historical events to particular views on AIDS, or to medical mistrust in general. The Tuskegee Study is a case in point. Reference to this study is almost *de rigueur* for any published work on the racial dimensions of AIDS conspiracy beliefs and medical mistrust. It is also often referred to in the black media. For example, in an editorial on Boyd Graves in *Cleveland Life*, the news editor wrote: "Is what Boyd Ed Graves saying accurate? I would respond with another question: If we would have been told about the experiments with blacks in Tuskegee with the syphilis virus, would we have believed the crier then?"[132] But for all its cultural importance, clear evidence as to how "Tuskegee" drives individual attitudes and behaviors is lacking. Studies have found that willingness to participate in biomedical research is unrelated to knowledge of the Tuskegee Study,[133] and that medical mistrust in the black community predates public disclosures about the Tuskegee Study[134] and is uncorrelated with knowledge of it.[135] Tuskegee is clearly important, but it is probably standing in for, or symbolic of, a structure of feeling that rests on a much wider experience than Tuskegee.

History and social context matter—but this is far from the only thing that determines whether particular individuals choose to endorse AIDS conspiracy beliefs or not. Individual psychologies, experiences, and social circumstances act to shape why some individuals in the same broad sociohistorical context find AIDS conspiracy beliefs compelling, whereas others do not. Chapter 3 considers this issue.

3

WHO BELIEVES AIDS CONSPIRACY THEORIES AND WHY LEADERSHIP MATTERS

C hapter 2 discussed the historical and political reasons why AIDS origin conspiracy theories are thinkable, but the fact that people in the same broad sociohistorical context differ in their embrace of them suggests that individual-level factors are also important. Exploring which individual characteristics are associated with AIDS conspiracy beliefs may help us understand why, and possibly how, they acquire social traction.

This chapter analyzes potential determinants of AIDS conspiracy beliefs among young adults in Cape Town. The key finding is that socioeconomic, demographic, cultural, and psychological characteristics matter, but that political allegiance (notably, trust in President Mbeki's health minister) was also strongly positively correlated with AIDS conspiracy beliefs. Those who had never heard of the Treatment Action Campaign (TAC), the civil society movement that opposed Mbeki's AIDS policies, were also more likely to believe AIDS conspiracy theories. These two findings indicate that political leadership is important—both from within and outside of the state—in shaping whether people find AIDS conspiracy beliefs credible or not. The chapter concludes with a reflection on how we should think about the problem of poor leadership, taking Louis Farrakhan's promotion of the ineffective AIDS drug Kemron as a US-based example.

RACE, GENDER, AND SOCIOECONOMIC STATUS

Table 3.1 shows that race is a key determinant of belief in AIDS origin conspiracy theories in South Africa, with black (African) people being far more likely than other population groups (white or mixed race) to endorse them. Whereas 16 percent of black survey respondents scored an average of "agree" on the AIDS conspiracy belief index, only 1 percent of the rest of the sample did so. Interestingly, AIDS conspiracy beliefs have a strongly gendered dimension in the black population (with men being significantly more likely to endorse them than women) but not among other groups.

That race is correlated with belief in AIDS origin conspiracies is unsurprising given the history of racially discriminatory medical abuse and biowarfare in South Africa (chapter 2). But why are there gender differences? In the most thorough ethnographic study available on AIDS conspiracy beliefs among black South Africans, Isak Niehaus and Gunvor Jonsson reported that men "variously identified right-wing whites, Dr. Wouter Basson, South Africa's governments, Americans, businesspeople and the military as sources of the epidemic," but that they encountered no such stories among women, even when asked directly about them.[1] They speculate that this may have to do with women being focused on a relatively secure local/domestic context (in which the state provides child-support grants) while men are more exposed (via the labor market) to international political-economic forces beyond their control.[2]

Their analysis thus suggests that income security and socioeconomic status may be relevant in shaping whether people believe AIDS conspiracy theories or not. In this regard, several US studies suggest that socioeconomic status may matter, but the statistical effects are small and often inconsistent.[3] In their survey of black churchgoers in the United States, Parsons and colleagues concluded that "each segment of African American society" was equally likely to believe AIDS conspiracies.[4] A broader

TABLE 3.1

AIDS ORIGIN CONSPIRACY BELIEFS
(YOUNG ADULTS, CAPE TOWN, AGED 19–29)

	DISAGREE	NEITHER / DON'T KNOW	AGREE
1. AIDS WAS INVENTED TO KILL BLACK PEOPLE			
Black men	54%	23%	23%
Black women	66%	24%	11%
Black total	61%	24%	16%
Others (white and mixed race)	92%	8%	1%
2. AIDS WAS CREATED BY SCIENTISTS IN AMERICA			
Black men	36%	40%	23%
Black women	60%	31%	10%
Black total	49%	35%	16%
Others (white and mixed race)	85%	12%	3%
3. AIDS WAS DELIBERATELY CREATED BY HUMANS			
Black men	37%	37%	25%
Black women	57%	25%	18%
Black total	49%	30%	21%
Others (white and mixed race)	69%	21%	10%
AIDS ORIGIN CONSPIRACY BELIEFS (INDEX OF QUESTIONS 1–3)*			
Black men	48%	29%	23%
Black women	63%	27%	10%
Black total	57%	28%	16%
Others (white and mixed race)	83%	16%	1%

Source: Cape Area Panel Survey data, 2009 (total sample = 2,901, of which 45% were African). Data set is available on request through the Center for Social Science Research at the University of Cape Town.

*Constructed by summing the scores on a five-point Likert scale ranging from 1 for "Strongly Disagree" to 5 for "Strongly Agree" and dividing by three. *Note:* The three measures factor together (Eigen value = 2/7; alpha = 0.85).

US survey of black households similarly found that income and age were unrelated to belief in AIDS conspiracies (though being a college graduate raised the likelihood of being a believer) and that the key predictor for men endorsing AIDS conspiracy beliefs was frequent experiences of racial discrimination, whereas for women it was "a strong preference for black culture and a culturally traditional black family."[5]

Given these findings, it makes sense to include race, household income, and a measure of being "culturally traditional" in our exploration of the South African data below. Given that the black South African sample was Xhosa-speaking, and that male circumcision is a strong Xhosa tradition (although some young people are beginning to challenge it),[6] the specific cultural indicator used was whether survey respondents agreed or disagreed with the statement that "a man is not really a man if he has not been through a traditional circumcision ceremony."

AGENCY PANIC, WITCHCRAFT, AND OTHER PSYCHO-SPIRITUAL CONCERNS

Psychological factors also need to be considered. When Richard Hofstadter coined the term "paranoid style" with regard to conspiracy theory, he did so to evoke "qualities of heated exaggeration, suspiciousness and conspiratorial fantasy" rather than suggesting it "applied only to people with profoundly disturbed minds."[7] But even though clinical paranoia is not a necessary condition for adopting a "paranoid style" toward AIDS conspiracy theory, it is nevertheless possible that people with "profoundly disturbed minds" are more prone to belief in conspiracy theories. Furthermore, as literary scholar Elaine Showalter has observed, conspiracy theories may be "cultural narratives of hysteria," arising out of a "universal psychopathology of everyday life."[8] This suggests that we ought to include a measure of psychological distress in our statistical exploration of who believes AIDS conspiracy theories. We do this by using the six-item "Kessler scale,"[9] which asks how often people experience nervousness, hopelessness, restlessness, depression, worthlessness, and the feeling that everything is an effort. Responses (ranging from 0 for "never," to 4 for "all of the time") are summed, with scores of 13 and more typically regarded as indicating severe psychological distress, even possible serious mental illness.[10]

A related concern is that some form of cognitive failure may play a role in whether people endorse conspiracy theories or not. This idea is evident in Hofstadter's observation that belief in conspiracy theory is perverse insofar as it requires a willingness to accept "a chain of deception so complex, an intelligence so formidable and a cast of accomplices so large (and silent) that the whole scheme collapses of its own implausibility."[11] Fredric Jameson makes a similar point when he describes conspiracy theory as a "poor person's cognitive mapping" and as a desperate and "degraded" attempt to represent the complex impersonal forces of late capitalism and the postmodern world.[12] More recent scholarship worries that such analysis is overly "pathologizing" and demonstrates a "patrician distaste" for conspiracy theory rather than seeking to understand its social origins and cultural logic.[13] Postmodernist Jodi Dean suggests that calling a conspiracy theory "distorted" merely reveals a "play of power, one often made on the part of a dominant group against those who may perceive themselves as threatened, marginalised, or oppressed."[14] Even so, it is nevertheless possible that *some* individuals may endorse conspiracy beliefs because of poor access to information or because they lack appropriate cognitive skills—even while recognizing that conspiracy beliefs *in general* should not be accounted for in this way.

Some analysts explain belief in AIDS conspiracy theories as a rational coping mechanism in the face of uncontrollable external forces.[15] This dovetails with cultural approaches emphasizing that people now live in situations fraught with risk and uncertainty,[16] where master narratives have been replaced by a multiplicity of meanings and where practices of the imagination are increasingly important.[17] Notably, Paula Treichler locates AIDS conspiracy beliefs within what she terms a broader "epidemic of signification" or parallel cultural process in which people generate, reproduce, and perform meanings in an attempt "to understand—however imperfectly—the complex, puzzling and quite terrifying phenomenon of AIDS."[18] In some interpretations, the process of constructing and believing conspiracy theories can be empowering insofar as it provides a framework for challenging an often oppressive hegemony and potentially uncovering real abuses of power.[19] Most, however, see it as indicative of powerlessness. Timothy Melley argues that conspiracy theories arises out of "agency panic" over a deeply felt loss of autonomy: "In moments of agency panic, individuals tend to attribute to these systems the qualities of motive, agency, and individuality they suspect have been depleted from themselves or others around them."[20]

Psychologists John Mirowsky and Catherine Ross argued in an influential piece that belief that one's life is being controlled by external forces, mistrust, and paranoia "form a stairway of deepening alienation" in which the individual "descends from a sense of powerlessness, or lack of control, to one of being used and abused, and finally, to one of being attacked."[21] They thus predicted (and found) a correlation between belief in external control, low socioeconomic status, and low levels of trust in others. However, US studies of AIDS conspiracy beliefs have come to contradictory findings in this respect. Some found that belief in conspiracies was associated with anomie, insecurity of employment, lack of interpersonal trust,[22] and with feelings of alienation, powerlessness, hostility, and being disadvantaged.[23] Others have found no correlation with socioeconomic status or psychological variables (such as powerlessness and tendency to attribute blame externally) and beliefs in US government conspiracies against black people.[24]

Melley's theory of "agency panic" is similar to the analysis of witchcraft beliefs as persisting in the modern world precisely because they speak to anxieties about the impersonal, powerful, and potentially harmful forces of global capitalism. As Edward Evans-Pritchard pointed out as early as 1937, witchcraft beliefs are able to provide meaning to undeserved, seemingly random suffering, by attributing it to the malicious intent of others.[25] Subsequent ethnography has shown that, far from fading away with modernity, witchcraft beliefs have proved highly adaptable to changing circumstances[26]—largely for this reason.

Todd Sanders and Harry West make a direct link between "occult cosmologies" (including witchcraft) and the world of conspiracy theory:

> Not only do occult cosmologies suggest that power sometimes hides itself from view, but they also often suggest that it conspires to fulfil its objectives (each an essential trait of conspiracy theories). In this way, oc-

cult cosmologies potentially contain within them theories of conspiracy. On the other side of the coin, although conspiracy theories are not necessarily fully-fledged cosmologies, they contain occult perspectives on the world, for they too, concern themselves with the operation of secret, mysterious and/or unseen powers. They too, suggest that there is more to power than meets the eye.[27]

There is a rich South African literature suggesting that many black people believe that HIV may have spiritual causes, notably witchcraft attacks or loss of protection from ancestors through violating cultural taboos.[28] As Adam Ashforth observes, "a disease or complex of symptoms better suited to interpretation within the witchcraft paradigm than AIDS would be harder to imagine."[29] This is because the symptoms of AIDS—diarrhea, tuberculosis, and wasting are also the classic symptoms of *isidliso*, or poisoning through witchcraft.[30] Thus, even where people accept that AIDS is caused by a sexually transmitted virus, suspicions of witchcraft may be retained as potential explanations for the ultimate reason behind the infection.[31]

But whether there is a link between belief in witchcraft as an ultimate (if not proximate) cause of AIDS and belief in AIDS conspiracy theories is an open empirical issue. Belief in AIDS conspiracies has been associated with the attribution of ill health to malevolent occult forces in Zimbabwe,[32] but there is no systematic research on exactly this connection in South Africa. Ashforth suggests that "within the witchcraft paradigm, the tendency is to presume that the secret source of power lying behind appearances is inherently evil" and that suspicion could eventually fall upon the state if nothing is done (against witches) to stop the suffering.[33] Such a scenario is consistent with the development of conspiracy theories about evil forces lurking within the state (or even in powerful foreign countries like the United States). Jonny Steinberg, however, hypothesizes that precisely because the very "idea that an epidemic of envy is killing the young and the healthy in large numbers is perhaps intolerable," people erect a "rickety fence" around HIV by claiming publicly that it is *not* caused by witchcraft[34]—even though many privately continue to harbor suspicions about it.

Anthropologist Max Marwick famously suggested that witchcraft functions as a "social strain gauge" whereby witchcraft accusations are likely to become more widespread in times of crisis.[35] An AIDS epidemic undoubtedly causes "social strain," and it is likely that the same factors (fear, uncertainty) which may prompt suspicions of witchcraft may also, for related reasons, prompt individuals to consider other potential sources of evil intent, notably AIDS conspiracy theories about evil scientists and Americans. Thus, for this reason too there may be an affinity between witchcraft beliefs and AIDS conspiracy theories, as both imply a hidden evil power and both are responses to very contemporary fears and conundrums pertaining to the AIDS epidemic. A variable to capture this particular worldview—namely, whether the respondent believes that witchcraft should "always" be suspected if a young person dies—is accordingly included in the statistical analysis below. Those who wish to skip the statistical analysis may skip directly to section 3.4, which opens with a brief summary of the findings.

LEADERSHIP AND OTHER DETERMINANTS OF AIDS CONSPIRACY BELIEFS IN CAPE TOWN: AN EXPLORATORY STATISTICAL ANALYSIS

Table 3.2 presents two models of AIDS conspiracy beliefs Eduard Grebe and I derived for young adults in Cape Town. They include variables to capture the effect of traditionalism, witchcraft beliefs, trust in others, social marginalization (whether people are employed or in supportive social structures such as religious organizations), and socioeconomic status, as well as the Kessler scale measure of psychological distress. By including these variables in a multivariate analysis that also attempts to capture the impact of political variables, it is possible to explore whether trust in Tshabalala-Msimang (Mbeki's health minister) mattered for AIDS conspiracy beliefs, and whether exposure to the TAC made any difference, after taking into account other relevant factors.

To explore trust in Tshabalala-Msimang, we measured whether respondents trusted her more than Barbara Hogan, the health minister who replaced her.[36] Both health ministers belonged to the same political party (the ANC), but as Hogan is white (whereas Tshabalala-Msimang was black), it is possible that relative trust in the two women was driven by racial, rather

TABLE 3.2

MODELING AIDS CONSPIRACY BELIEFS

DEPENDENT VARIABLE: SCORE OF "AGREE" OR "STRONGLY AGREE" ON THE AIDS CONSPIRACY BELIEF INDEX (SEE TABLE 3.1)	FULL SAMPLE	BLACK SOUTH AFRICANS
	MODEL 1	MODEL 2
Black (African)	6.71***	
	(1.81)	
Female	0.89	0.91
	(0.16)	(0.20)
Any tertiary education	0.68	0.45**
	(0.17)	(0.14)
Household income per capita (log)	0.81***	0.77***
	(0.07)	(0.08)
Seriously psychologically distressed (Kessler psychological distress scale > 12)	2.92***	2.96***
	(0.61)	(0.71)
Trust Mbeki's health minister more than her successor	2.99***	3.98***
	(0.52)	(0.82)
Attitude to blacks minus attitude to whites	1.10***	1.13***
	(0.03)	(0.37)
Never heard of TAC	1.89***	1.79**
	(0.35)	(0.40)
Often gets news from radio/TV/newspaper	1.11	1.0
	(0.18)	(0.19)
Member of a religious organization	0.67**	0.57***
	(0.12)	(0.12)
Agrees a man is not a man until he has		3.10***
		(1.12)
Agrees witchcraft should always be suspected when a young person dies		3.36***
		(0.96)
Observations	1,886	1.115
Pseudo R^2	0.20	0.21

*$p < 0.10$, **$p < 0.05$, ***$p < 0.01$. Other independent variables included were age, school grades completed, employment status, and whether respondents agree that most people can be trusted or voted in the last election. These socioeconomic variables and measures of potential social alienation were included as controls, but proved not to be statistically significant and thus were not reported for brevity's sake. For more details, see Grebe and Nattrass (2011). Data from Cape Area Panel Survey (see table 3.1).

than AIDS-related, concerns. To address this potentially confounding factor, a further variable is included measuring the difference between the respondent's scores on a social distance scale for black people and white people: the larger the value, the more the respondent "likes" blacks relative to whites.

A second political variable attempts to capture the influence of the TAC in resisting the Mbeki government's approach to AIDS. The TAC, whose membership is primarily black and poor, aligned itself with the black trade unions and the predominantly white medical profession to promote the scientific consensus on HIV prevention and treatment. This broad alliance cut across racial and class divides to challenge Mbeki and Tshabalala-Msimang's political authority on AIDS and their attempts to racialize AIDS policy. The TAC organized public protests, conducted various legal actions, and engaged in substantial AIDS information and treatment literacy campaigns.[37] To capture the influence of the TAC, we include a variable ("never heard of the TAC"), which takes a value of 1 if the respondents indicated that they have never heard of the organization (and a value of 0 if they have). As this variable could be a proxy for whether the respondent is generally well informed or not, we included a further control variable taking a value of 1 if respondents reported that they "often" obtained news from the radio or newspapers or television.

Table 3.2 presents two (logistic) regressions on AIDS conspiracy beliefs—measured as whether the respondent registered as agreeing or agreeing strongly on the AIDS conspiracy index reported in table 3.1. The first figure in each cell is an odds ratio reporting the effect of the variable on the odds of endorsing AIDS conspiracies. Thus, the first variable reported in Model 1 (which is run on the total sample) tells us that after taking into account the effects of the other variables, the odds of believing AIDS conspiracies rises by a factor of 6.71 (i.e., almost sevenfold) if the respondent is black. This is highly statistically significant as evidenced by the low p-value (three stars) and low standard error.[38]

Model 2 is run on black respondents only and includes the two specifically African cultural variables. Both models show that the gender differences suggested in table 3.1 are statistically insignificant and that what appeared to be a gender difference is accounted for by other variables. People living in more financially secure households were less likely to endorse AIDS conspiracy theories, and black respondents with a tertiary education were less than half as likely to endorse AIDS conspiracy theories. None of the other demographic and socioeconomic variables (school grades completed, employment status, and age) were statistically significant in either model.

By contrast, being seriously psychologically distressed almost tripled the odds of endorsing AIDS conspiracy beliefs in both models. Does this mean that psychological distress renders people more likely to believe in AIDS conspiracy theories? Perhaps. The point to bear in mind is that this sort of analysis can only establish correlation—not the direction of causation. It may well be that causality runs in the opposite direction, i.e., that belief in conspiracy theories about the origin of AIDS itself causes mental distress. After all, to believe that doctors and scientists are colluding to hide the truth about HIV being a bioweapon, and that they may actually be out to kill Africans with their tests and drugs, must have distressing implications for how people feel about the world and their place in it. To quote Hofstadter once more: "We are all sufferers from history, but the paranoid is a double sufferer, since he is afflicted not only by the real world, with the rest of us, but by his fantasies as well."[39]

Interestingly, being a member of a religious organization significantly reduced the odds of endorsing conspiracy theories—especially for black South Africans. This may be because people who find themselves attracted to AIDS conspiracy theories are also the kind of people who find religion compelling, perhaps even necessary, given their fearful beliefs about evil medical practitioners and the like. Or it may be because religiously inspired attitudes toward AIDS (for example, that it is a punishment from God) act as counter-narratives to AIDS conspiracy beliefs.[40]

Traditional cultural attitudes, by contrast, are strongly positively associated with belief in AIDS conspiracy theories among black South Africans. Model 2 shows that after taking into account the influence of the other variables in the model, belief that a man is not a man until he has been through the circumcision ritual triples the odds of also endorsing AIDS conspiracy theories. A similar finding is evident for belief in witchcraft.[41] As the direction of causality is unlikely to run from AIDS conspiracy beliefs to holding culturally traditional attitudes, this suggests that those with more traditional cultural beliefs are also more likely to believe AIDS conspiracy theories than others.

Another significant and substantive determinant of belief in AIDS conspiracies was whether respondents trusted Tshabalala-Msimang more than her successor. It shows that controlling for other variables (including racial preferences) those who trusted Tshabalala-Msimang more than Hogen were three times as likely to believe AIDS conspiracy theories (Model 1) and four times as likely if they were black (Model 2). This suggests that Mbeki and Tshabalala-Msimang either directly influenced public support for AIDS conspiracy beliefs or at least reinforced them by playing to an already existing openness toward AIDS conspiracy beliefs among Mbeki's supporters.

The role of the TAC also appears to have been important. Controlling for other variables (including whether respondents were generally well informed or not), the odds of believing AIDS conspiracy theories almost doubled for respondents who had never heard of the TAC. This suggests that the scientific approach to AIDS adopted by the TAC may have undermined the credibility of rival conspiracy accounts.[42]

That trust in political leaders and challenges from civil society matter for AIDS conspiracy beliefs highlights the importance of political leadership, both from within government and in civil society. Although we cannot know for sure whether it was the fact that respondents trusted Tshabalala-Msimang that made them more likely to believe AIDS conspiracy theories, or whether it was their prior belief in AIDS origin conspiracies which encouraged them to trust her, the fact that there was a correlation between these two variables tells us at least that there is a strong intersection between political allegiance and AIDS conspiracy beliefs.

We can, however, feel more certain about the direction of causality with regard to knowledge of the TAC. The question posed was a neutral one—simply whether respondents had ever heard of the TAC, not whether they trusted or supported it. That those who had never heard of the TAC were more likely to believe AIDS origin conspiracies suggests that the TAC has been able to combat AIDS conspiracy beliefs, presumably through its treatment literacy programs and active contestation of Mbeki and Tshabalala-

Msimang's policies. Taken together, this suggests that had the government accepted and promoted the scientific consensus on AIDS, we may well have had fewer AIDS conspiracy believers today.

IMPLICATIONS FOR HOW WE UNDERSTAND AIDS CONSPIRACY BELIEFS

In sum, the above analysis suggests that AIDS conspiracy believers in Cape Town are more likely to be black, psychologically distressed, to trust Mbeki's health minister more than her successor, to never have heard of the TAC, and not to be members of a religious organization. They are also likely to come from poorer households and, in the case of black South Africans, not to have any tertiary education or to have voted in the last election. Black respondents who believe in witchcraft and who hold traditional values (at least as far as the link between masculinity and circumcision is concerned) are also more likely to endorse AIDS conspiracy theories.

This suggests that the picture is socioeconomically, culturally, and psychologically complex. And, as the models account for less than a quarter of the total variation in the answers, it is important to note that there are lots of missing factors from our explanation. Even so, the results suggest that hypotheses about conspiracy beliefs being a response to social and economic marginalization may be on to something, at least in this sample of young adults from Cape Town.

Cultural beliefs also seem to matter, though precisely in what way is unclear. Consider the witchcraft variable. Does the correlation between belief that witchcraft should be suspected if a young person dies and AIDS conspiracy belief mean that conspiracy beliefs and witchcraft beliefs are part of a broader cultural form in which evil forces are assumed to be widespread and powerful in shaping the affairs of humankind? Or is it picking up a general level of anxiety about AIDS deaths and socioeconomic insecurity (the social strain interpretation)? The same conundrum applies to the variable capturing psychological distress, as we do not know the extent to which this variable is capturing mental illness, or distress that is caused by AIDS, unemployment, and perhaps even belief in conspiracies themselves.

Considering the fluid nature of AIDS conspiracy beliefs (discussed in chapter 2) and the contingent and complex psycho-social-cultural factors highlighted by the statistical analysis here, it probably makes sense simply to conclude that the reasons why people endorse AIDS origin conspiracy beliefs are likely to differ at the individual level, even for those with similar historical and socioeconomic backgrounds. The wider cultural and historical context makes AIDS origin conspiracies thinkable, but the decision to embrace them is an individual one fraught with complexities pertaining to personality, education, attitudes, and political engagement.

What does this mean for how we should understand people's beliefs in AIDS conspiracy theories? Medical anthropologist and physician Paul Farmer argues that people should be treated as "experts in a moral reading of the ills that afflict them" and analysts should "extend a 'hermeneutic of generosity' to the very notions dismissed as paranoid rubbish by the experts."[43] Triechler makes the point more strongly when she adopts the subaltern voice to argue that "we cannot afford to let scientists or any other group of experts dismiss our meanings as 'misconceptions' and our alternative views as noise that interferes with the pure processes of scientific enquiry."[44] While their cautions are important, the terrain is much more complex than a putative struggle between "experts" and alternative views. Treichler's use of "our" (implying the notion of a collective "we") is problematic in that it assumes uniformity and avoids confronting the issue that some voices are more powerful and influential than others. It is not enough to depict AIDS conspiracy beliefs simply as counter-narratives or rival ways of knowing: we need to ask who promotes these views, how are they supported, and do they cause harm.

Consider the role of Mbeki and Tshabalala-Msimang. The analysis presented in this chapter suggests a connection between their political influence and belief in AIDS conspiracies. Given that these beliefs undermine safe sex,[45] this poses an ongoing problem for fighting the HIV epidemic. Chapter 5 looks at the South African story in more detail, arguing that Mbeki exercised an even greater impact on the epidemic by delaying the use of antiretrovirals for either mother-to-child transmission prevention or AIDS treatment. It was not Mbeki who was the powerless voice here. It was the tens of thousands of babies who contracted HIV unnecessarily and the hundreds of thousands of people who died from AIDS untreated who were the truly marginalized, subaltern voices. Furthermore, his views were idiosyncratic and strongly opposed—as evidenced by the successful political struggle waged against him. Under these circumstances, analyzing Mbeki's stance as emblematic of some legitimate alternative popular counter-narrative to expert opinion is not only misleading but runs the danger of sliding into apologetics. For example, French anthropologist Didier Fassin presents Mbeki's approach to AIDS as an understandable African reaction to Western discourses of blame and to the way biomedical approaches neglect the role of poverty in driving the HIV epidemic.[46] In Fassin's sympathetic account, Mbeki was expressing the will of millions of aggrieved compatriots in the face of a hostile and arrogant AIDS establishment. But as Steinberg points out, not only does this ignore the fact that Mbeki was politically isolated within his own party and unable to win mass support for his policies, but it effectively condemned all Africans via his "anthropology of low expectations":

> Fassin is quick to talk Mbeki up as the voice of a resonant African experience and a powerful African nationalism. And yet in doing so, he comes close to saying that African nationalism was destined to get the aetiology of AIDS horribly wrong. Berating the orthodox for their blindness to the anguish of the vanquished, he is on the brink of saying that we must expect nothing more from African nationalism than resentment and suspicion.[47]

These issues are taken up again in chapter 5. At this point, suffice to say that leadership, influence, and strategies for constructing credibility matter and ought to matter for how we think about the social dimensions of AIDS origin conspiracy beliefs. The strong link between trust in Mbeki's health minister relative to her successor is indicative of the powerful role that politicians are able to play in both promoting and contesting AIDS conspiracy theories. As our results for the influence of the TAC suggest, leadership from the community level can also play an influential role in contesting and undermining AIDS conspiracy beliefs. But community leadership is not always as progressive. As discussed below with regard to the United States, charismatic community leadership can promote, rather than contest, AIDS conspiracy beliefs.

POOR COMMUNITY LEADERSHIP:
THE CASE OF FARRAKHAN AND KEMRON

How can we simultaneously critique political leaders for their stance on AIDS—while also seeking to understand the historical context that gives rise to it? In her discussion of the African-American community's response to AIDS, sociologist Cathy Cohen usefully distinguishes between "primary marginalization," i.e., the socioeconomic and institutional disadvantages faced by African-Americans, and "secondary marginalization" resulting from the "exercise of power by more privileged marginal group members over others in their community."[48] In Cohen's account, the African-American elite and media in the 1980s and 1990s failed the broader black community because they were primarily concerned to portray African-Americans as respectable and successful, and that AIDS conspiracy theories assisted this project by attributing HIV to external sources and deflecting attention away from the politically difficult challenge of addressing risk behaviors within the community. As she observes dryly, "rarely do these stories of conspiracy call for the mobilisation of black communities around the issue. Instead, readers are encouraged to be personally outraged and satisfied with uncovering another deadly plot on the part of government conspirators."[49]

By acknowledging that AIDS conspiracy theories gained legitimacy because they resonated with "a deserved mistrust of the government among African-Americans,"[50] but then going on to problematize the role of leaders for their failure to challenge (and sometimes even their active promotion of), these theories, Cohen shows that it is possible to combine contextual analysis with critique. She provides herself with the space for robust criticism of leaders and opinion-makers for their contribution to the secondary marginalization of people at risk of HIV in the community.

Consider the case of Kemron, the ineffective AIDS drug heavily promoted by some leaders and opinion-makers in the African-American community—most notably by Louis Farrakhan, the charismatic head of the Nation of Islam.[51] Cohen's distinction allows us to acknowledge that enthusiasm within the African-American community for this supposed African cure resonated within a particular historical and socioeconomic context of primary marginalization, but that by making further conspiratorial moves against medical science while promoting Kemron in its place, Farrakhan contributed to the secondary marginalization of vulnerable people within the community.

Kemron hit the headlines in 1990 when Davy Koech and Arthur Obel from the Kenyan Medical Research Institute (KEMRI) published results from a flawed clinical trial (which lacked a control group), claiming that low-dose oral alpha interferon improved the health of AIDS patients and even resulted in some patients "sero-reverting" to HIV-negative status.[52] HIV scientists elsewhere were skeptical, not only because of the trial design but because injected doses of oral alpha interferon 10,000 times higher had by this time been shown to be ineffective,[53] and a subsequent review by the National Institutes of Health (NIH) of the thirteen studies of alpha interferon concluded that patients were better off not taking it.[54] But the drug was heavily promoted in the African-American community in a discourse laden with suspicion. As a report put it:

> Harlem physician Barbara Justice visited KEMRI and extolled Kemron on her weekly radio health show on WLIB-AM, a New York station with a black nationalist orientation. New York's *Amsterdam News* and the *Washington Afro-American* regularly criticized the NIH for ignoring the KEMRI results and helped spread the theory that a racist conspiracy by white researchers was suppressing the discovery.[55]

Farrakhan continued to pressure the NIH for a new US-based trial[56] while offering a very expensive version of Kemron (selling at $1,500 at a time when a New York buyers club was providing it for $50 and then eventually just giving it away)[57] to AIDS patients through Nation of Islam clinics. The Nation of Islam's publication *Final Call* also promoted conspiracy theories about the man-made origins of AIDS, claiming that FDA-approved antiretrovirals were poisonous and part of a white conspiracy to kill African-Americans.[58] Such pressure eventually paid off and the NIH agreed to conduct a further US-based trial—despite opposition from HIV scientists and AIDS activists, including Martin Delaney of Project Inform.[59] A *Newsweek* story on the "angry politics of Kemron" concluded that the trial was necessary for political reasons: "By ignoring the Kemron outcry, the government would only harden the suspicion that it is suppressing a treatment that works. In purely scientific terms, there may be more promising drugs to investigate. But where AIDS is concerned, science has to accommodate the world."[60]

The trial was initiated (including through Nation of Islam clinics—despite the obvious conflict of interest)[61] but eventually stopped in the mid-1990s because of insufficient enrollment. By this time, highly active antiretroviral treatment (HAART) had been shown to be effective and the Kenyan patients who had been previously been declared "cured" of HIV by Koech and Obel were suing them in court.[62] This, however, did not deter the Nation of Islam, which continued to promote the drug.[63] Farrakhan was reportedly still promoting the drug as late as 2002, even offering Kemron to President Robert Mugabe.[64] That Farrakhan was both promoting AIDS conspiracy beliefs and a putative cure for AIDS places him firmly within the ranks of the cultropreneurs.

The powerful synergistic connection between AIDS conspiracy theories, rejection of scientifically proven therapies, and the promotion of alternative cures is evident in this following account by LeRoy Whitfield, the *POZ* magazine journalist who interviewed Boyd Graves for his investigation into AIDS conspiracy theories in the African-American community (see chapter 2). Whitfield reports how, as an HIV-positive man, he was at first enthralled by the package Farrakhan had to offer:

> Bow-tied and freshly dipped in an Italian suit, he [Farrakhan] stepped up to a mike in the fall of 1992 at a downtown Chicago hotel. . . . Farrakhan's message was loud and clear. If you're taking AZT, he told the audience, ditch it—it's poisonous. That's possible, I thought, considering all the rumors of 'hood deaths I'd heard. And HIV, he went on, was created in a government lab in Virginia. Son of a bitch, I thought, my life's been turned

upside-down as a result of covert government warfare. And considering the dehumanizing government-run Tuskegee syphilis experiment—just halted in 1972, three years after I was born—Big Lou's idea didn't seem so far-fetched to me. But here's the clincher: The good minister then revealed to us that a Kenyan doctor had discovered an AIDS cure: Kemron. The word cure spoke directly to my soul. . . . What Minister Farrakhan was offering, to my mind, wasn't just alternative medication but sorely needed liberation. To hell with trying to understand HIV or ever being a slave to oddball medical regimen, I thought. I am free.[65]

Whitfield goes on to report that his hopes for Kemron were soon dashed once he investigated further. Unfortunately, though, he could never bring himself to take antiretroviral treatment and died of kidney failure and pneumonia.

Was Farrakhan promoting Kemron because it was an African cure? Delaney thought not, pointing out that the oral alpha interferon cure had surfaced originally in the United States. The idea that oral alpha interferon might benefit AIDS patients was initially conceived by Joseph Cummins, a veterinarian from Texas, who used it to treat cattle.[66] It was he who provided Koech and the Nation of Islam with powdered versions of the drug. As Delaney angrily observed, although Farrakhan and his organization "pitched it as a 'black solution for AIDS,'" they "knew damned well where it came from." For this veteran AIDS activist, Farrakhan was simply "beyond redemption."[67]

But the secondary marginalization of vulnerable African-Americans by Farrakhan fades in comparison to that experienced by South Africans under Mbeki. Chapter 5 takes a closer look at Mbeki's contestation of HIV science and at the human consequences of the delayed rollout of antiretrovirals for HIV prevention and treatment. It concludes that AIDS policy failures can be laid largely at the door of AIDS denialism and associated conspiratorial moves against science. But before delving into this story, chapter 4 concludes the focus on AIDS origin conspiracy theories by exploring how political and scientific arguments were mobilized by a trusted peer-educator in the US prison system to counter them.

4

SCIENCE, POLITICS, AND CREDIBILITY

DAVID GILBERT FIGHTS AIDS CONSPIRACY BELIEFS IN US PRISONS

David Gilbert is a prisoner who cofounded a peer AIDS education initiative in response to rising rates of HIV infection and AIDS deaths in US prisons during the late 1980s and early 1990s.[1] Most interestingly for our purposes, as part of this effort he penned an influential article debunking the conspiracy theory that HIV had been manufactured in a laboratory. Gilbert argued that although there were good reasons why people might suspect a laboratory origin for HIV, scientific evidence renders this theory implausible. In his account, the "real" genocidal aspect of the epidemic is the way discriminatory policies and exploitative socioeconomic structures make it more likely that vulnerable people will contract HIV and die of AIDS. As this is the most cogent and widely cited rebuttal of AIDS origin conspiracy theories, and because it has been subjected to a postmodern critique (by Jack Bratich), his analysis is of interest at both practical and theoretical levels.

Gilbert's motivation for taking on the claims of AIDS conspiracy theorists was that he had noticed that "those who most pushed AIDS conspiracy theories least discussed prevention."[2] This casual but important observation, borne out of long discussions with prisoners, is consistent with subsequent US studies showing an association between belief in AIDS conspiracy theories and failure to take steps to prevent HIV infection.[3] The same trend is evident in Cape Town, where a survey of young adults revealed that controlling for other determinants of sexual behavior, belief in AIDS conspiracy theories reduces the odds of using a condom by about a third.[4] There is, in short, substantial evidence on both sides of the Atlantic that the conspiratorial move against HIV science tends to be accompanied by the rejection of mainstream messages about how HIV is transmitted and prevented.

Yet it took a while for scholars to grapple with the import of AIDS conspiracy beliefs, and even when this was done, very little attention was paid to critiquing them. Instead, analysts typically pointed to the understandable historical context for these beliefs while calling (vaguely) for culturally sensitive responses. David Gilbert, in the meantime, waited for an article to be produced that could assist him in his prison-based AIDS education activities, but when none was forthcoming, he eventually wrote it himself. Commenting on its enduring status as the classic critique of AIDS conspiracy theory, Gilbert wrote to me saying:

> I feel honored that you highlight my work, but at the same time chagrined that evidently there haven't been subsequent works that are more thorough and more persuasive. That's especially so because 6 months later, I could have done the scientific argument in a stronger way—but when I wrote I had already procrastinated for 6 years, waiting for someone in a better position to do a better job, for something so lethal.[5]

Why were academics reluctant to grapple with and critique AIDS origin conspiracy theories? Perhaps the problem was that the connection between these beliefs and risky behavior had yet to be firmly established. Perhaps it was a general reluctance to take on what were perceived to be obviously crank theories circulating in the cultic milieu. But it is also likely that the "postmodern turn" in the social sciences encouraged scholars to concentrate on the rhetorical strategies employed by those making truth claims, rather than to take a stance on the truth claims themselves. Thus, for example,

Jack Bratich argues that "rather than accept conspiracy theories as a real danger to the health of the body politic," we should rather "ask how the risky thought encapsulated in the conspiracy theory problem is generated discursively" (but in so doing, he ends up making truth claims of his own by calling arguments about the harm caused by conspiracy belief "conspiracy panics").[6]

Discourse analysts typically adopt relativist positions on conspiracy theories. For example, John Fiske argues that "we will never know 'objectively' whether or not AIDS is part of a genocidal strategy, for any evidence that might establish such a truth will be 'lost' or, should it survive, be strenuously denied."[7] He thus approaches AIDS origin conspiracy theory simply as a "counterknowledge," a practice of resistance in which various facts, events, and information, some of them dismissed by the "dominant knowledge," are "rearticulated into a counter way of knowing, where their significance is quite different."[8] Jack Bratich uses a similar approach to criticize David Gilbert for acknowledging science's "dirty history"—i.e., involvement in biowarfare and medical abuse—while simultaneously accepting the veracity of scientific evidence on AIDS. For Bratich, this is an unacceptable rhetorical move because it assumes "that we know when science was/is impure (mixed with power, used as a weapon) and when it is pure (as method, as official history)." He goes on to say: "A critic might counter that by not respecting the distinction [between science as a weapon of abuse and science as method] we move dangerously close to throwing the baby out with the bathwater. However, this already presumes the distinction: It is more analogous to say the difficulty lies in distinguishing the dirty from the clean water in the bath before throwing it out."[9]

The problem with this relativist philosophical stance is that it ends up assuming, in effect, that the "HIV as bioweapon" theory is as plausible as HIV science. This may be intellectually neat, but precisely because it avoids making judgments about which "ways of knowing" are more credible, it is a highly constrained form of analysis with little practical value. Furthermore, to draw an equivalence between AIDS conspiracy theories and HIV science because AIDS conspiracy theories are unfalsifiable and because some scientists have been involved in bioweapons programs and unethical research practices is itself a rhetorical move which excuses the analyst from having to confront the very issue of weighing the credibility of rival claims and coming to reasoned judgments about them.

Just because real conspiracies exist does not mean that all conspiracy theories should be treated as equally valid. As Gilbert observes:

> We complained about (and were called "paranoid" about) COINTELPRO well before it was exposed; similarly with what was revealed in the Pentagon Papers. There are often conspiracies (although the ones that work and have a lasting effect are the ones that serve broader ruling class interests.). But that broad observation doesn't validate the range of cockamamie theories out there.[10]

To return to Brian Keeley's useful distinction with regard to conspiracy theories (page 3), cockamamie theories may be "logically possible," but many are literally "incredible." Consider for a moment what the rival accounts of HIV's origin require us to believe. In order to accept the scientific consensus on HIV, we are required to accept as credible the peer-reviewed research showing that HIV originated from SIV in Africa long before the special cancer virus program operated at Fort Detrick, long before genetic cloning had been developed, and thus long before scientists even had the capacity to manufacture new viruses. To accept AIDS origin conspiracy theories, however, we have to believe that scientific research on the link between SIV and HIV is fraudulent, that HIV was deliberately manufactured to cause harm, and that hundreds of thousands of researchers and health care professionals are participating in an elaborate sham to cover this up. To regard these claims as equivalent rival "counterknowledges" involves an incredible suspension of judgment.

Gilbert's approach was to engage with the underlying political reasons for the mistrust in HIV science—that many of his fellow inmates believed, and with good reason, that shadowy forces within the US government may have manufactured HIV to harm African-Americans. By stressing that his scientific source had a good civil rights record, whereas the author of the most popular AIDS conspiracy theory circulating in prison had dubious right-wing connections, Gilbert was able to cut through the political suspicions that rendered AIDS conspiracy theory believable. Bratich, however, claims that Gilbert was really engaging in a form of identity politics in which conspiracy theory was "articulated" to the political right as part of an effort to situate "the Left" within the dominant paradigm of science and reason. The contrasting positions are discussed in more detail below.

DAVID GILBERT CONTESTS AIDS CONSPIRACY BELIEFS IN PRISON

David Gilbert is currently serving three consecutive life sentences for his part in the 1981 "Brinks robbery" in which two police officers and a guard were killed. This was an operation of the Revolutionary Armed Task Force (RATF), a joint effort of a unit of the Black Liberation Army (BLA)—a clandestine outgrowth of the Black Panthers—and some allied white revolutionaries (like Gilbert). Gilbert, who was not at the scene of the robbery or involved in the shooting, was sentenced under the Felony Murder Law, which determines that all people involved in an action leading to murder are held legally responsible for it. Kuwasi Balagoon, a BLA activist involved in the same action, subsequently died in jail in December 1986—prompting Gilbert and two other friends of Balagoon to start an AIDS peer-education program the following year.[11]

Gilbert has a long track record of working with Marxist and radical black organizations. He joined the Congress of Racial Equality in 1962 (at age 17), and in 1965, as a university student, helped found the Columbia University chapter of Students for a Democratic Society (SDS), where he developed a reputation as an organizer and a Marxist theorist. When SDS split in 1969, Gilbert joined what became the Weather Underground, its purpose being to wage armed struggle in support of the Black Panthers and to oppose the Vietnam War by "bringing the war home." The Weather Underground conducted a campaign of bombings and jailbreaks in the early 1970s, but lost momentum after the end of the Vietnam War, finally disintegrating in 1977. Gilbert, however, went back underground in 1979, choosing to continue his revolutionary activities through the RATF.[12]

Gilbert's political background is relevant in understanding the credibility of his voice as a peer educator. Not only was his sympathy with black political causes clear, but his refusal to testify against his co-accused (a practice incentivized by the Felony Murder Law) meant that, at least as Gilbert saw it, his fellow prisoners could be confident he was "not a snitch."[13] His Marxist ideological background is also helpful in understanding his views about the "real" AIDS genocide (that it is rooted in socioeconomic marginalization and racist policies) and his openness toward the idea that the state is eminently capable of creating bioweapons and employing dirty tactics against perceived enemies both foreign and domestic.

Dan Berger, who interviewed Gilbert for his book *Outlaws of America: The Weather Underground and the Politics of Solidarity*, talks about a defining moment for Gilbert in February 1965 when, after reading about the sustained US bombing of Vietnam on the train into Harlem, Gilbert arrived at the home of a black child he was tutoring:

> "I can't believe it, our government is bombing people on the other side of the globe for no good reason" he remembers telling the mother of his student when she asked him what was troubling him. . . . Her response was immediate: "Bombing people for no good reason huh? Must be colored people who live there." Her comment connected the dots for Gilbert. "She made the connection in a very direct way that I had had trouble seeing, even though I had been working on both fronts (civil rights and peace) for some four years," he says. "I was still blinded by defining our system as a 'democracy' (with some faults) while she understood it as, in its essence, a racist and exploitative system."[14]

The process of "connecting the dots" is a central practice for conspiracy theorists. But in Gilbert's case, his Marxist view of the world prioritized systemic forces in which racism exacerbated economic exploitation rather than political conspiracies *per se*. Importantly, though, he was able to recognize early on how conspiratorial discourses and narratives within the black community were often symbolic, as representative of a structure of feeling rather than firmly held beliefs about specific conspiracies. This, in turn, shaped the way he responded to AIDS origin conspiracy beliefs: by explicitly recognizing why they are thinkable and then trying to persuade his audience that they were nevertheless mistaken in accepting them as true.

Gilbert's piece, originally titled "Tracking the Real Genocide: AIDS—Conspiracy or Unnatural Disaster?,"[15] was published in 1996 as the lead article (and on the front cover) of *Covert Action Quarterly*, and subsequently in his collected writings, *No Surrender: Writings from an Anti-Imperialist Political Prisoner*.[16] Arguing that there was an "almost perfect fit" between AIDS, social oppression, and "the extensive body of history of chemical and biological warfare (CBW) and medical experiments against people of color, prisoners, and other unsuspecting citizens," Gilbert confirms that "there are good reasons" why people believe that "government scientists deliberately created AIDS as a tool of genocide" (129–31). But he then adds:

> There is only one problem with this almost perfect fit: It is not true. The theories on how HIV—the virus that causes AIDS—was purposely spliced together in the laboratory wilt under scientific scrutiny. Moreover, these conspiracy theories divert energy from the work that must be done in the trenches if marginalized communities are to survive this epidemic: grassroots mobilization for AIDS prevention, and better care for people living with HIV. (Gilbert 2004:131)

In countering AIDS origin conspiracy beliefs, Gilbert adopts a two-pronged strategy by arguing that they are both scientifically implausible and politically dubious. He reports that he sent the first AIDS origin conspiracy theory he encountered (an article based on the Soviet-Stasi-Segal misinformation campaign—see chapter 2) to a professor of molecular genetics and microbiology who was also a long-standing friend from his civil rights and antiwar days. He says "while that does not make her analysis infallible, there is certainly no way she could be a conscious part of a conspiracy against oppressed people" (133). He reports that her "response to the article I had found so politically credible was unequivocal: the splice theory that the Segals' posit is scientifically impossible." Subsequent versions of the splice theory he sent to her met with the same fate: "none of the viruses posited in the various splice theories has nearly enough similarity (or homology) with HIV to be one of its parents" (133). This, he argues, together with the "lack of knowledge of any human retroviruses before the late 1970s and the compelling evidence for the earlier genesis of HIV virtually eliminate the possibility that scientists deliberately designed such a germ to destroy the human immune system" (135).

Bratich, however, criticizes Gilbert for investing "trust in the official record of science's history rather than the institutional secrecy endemic to CBW scientific practice" and for employing a rhetorical strategy that used "science's power to authorize his own position."[17] Note that in so doing, Bratich rejects Gilbert's stated motivations and descriptions of the intellectual process he went through in favor of his own *assumption* that Gilbert had started out with "a position" which he was trying to "authorize" by appealing to science. He was, in other words, making a factual claim, about Gilbert, at the center of an analysis which supposedly eschews truth claims. Gilbert, in turn, found it "strange that Bratich posits that I—of all people— would want such establishment legitimacy or think I could be the one to achieve it"[18] and, as discussed below, reacted angrily to Bratich's interpretation of his (Gilbert's) "real" political motivations.

Gilbert focused the bulk of his attention on William Campbell Douglass's theory that HIV is a communist-controlled US bioweapon spread through vaccination campaigns and even casual contact.[19] He does so because, in his experience as an AIDS educator, this theory was directly associated with risky behavior:

> I've been doing AIDS education in prison for over nine years; these conspiracy myths have proven to be the main internal obstacle—in terms of prisoner's consciousness—to concentrating on thorough and detailed work on risk reduction. What's the use, believers ask, of making all the hard choices to avoid spreading or contracting the disease if the government is going to find a way to infect people anyway? And what's the point of all the hassles of safer sex, or all the inconvenience of not sharing needles, if HIV can be spread, as many conspiracy theorists claim, by casual contact, such as sneezing or handling dishes?
>
> The core of the mind-set that undermines prevention efforts is "denial." People whose activities put them at risk are often so petrified that they don't even want to think about it. Conspiracy theories serve up a hip and

seemingly militant rationale for not confronting one's own risk practices. At the same time, such theories provide an apparently simple and satisfying alternative to the complex challenge of dealing with the myriad of social, behavioral, and medical factors that propel the epidemic.[20]

Gilbert also points out that Douglass had "become a prime source for many Black community militants and prisoners who embrace the conspiracy theory out of a sincere desire to fight genocide (135). It is with this particular audience in mind that he highlights the right-wing connections of conspiracy theorists like Douglass:

> We live in a strange and dangerous period when the attractive mantle of "militant anti-government movement" has been bestowed on ultra-right-wing, white supremacist groups. The only reason they can get away with such a farce is that their big brother—the police state—did such an effective job in the blood-soaked repression of the genuine opposition, such as the Black Panthers, rooted in the needs and aspirations of oppressed people. With people's movements silenced, the right has co-opted the critique of big government and big business to achieve new credibility. (Gilbert 2004:142)

He warns his readers about Douglass's anticommunist, anti-immigration, and anti–civil rights politics (140–42) and his links to "conscious racist forces" which may be behind some of the disinformation.[21] Bratich, however, interprets Gilbert's focus on Douglass as a deliberate strategy to "articulate" (i.e., link) AIDS origin conspiracy to the political Right while placing the Left "squarely within the dominant regime of truth where science and authority subdue competing subjugated claims."[22]

I sent Gilbert a copy of Bratich's argument (Bratich had never engaged with Gilbert, so this was the first he had heard of it). He replied as follows:

> the biggest difference between me and Bratich is that he is evidently a Prof. putting forward an esoteric position on theories of how knowledge develops in society—whereas I was writing as an AIDS activist in the trenches fighting a lethal epidemic. . . . He postulates my purpose was to position

the Left squarely within the dominant regime of truth, science, authority. No such thought ever occurred to me; in fact my bias was toward believing AIDS conspiracy theories when I first heard them. My urgent and overriding purpose was to understand the truth in order to SAVE LIVES. My secondary goal was to take on this new trend of irrational and harmful analysis perpetrated on the oppressed.[23] (emphasis in the original)

Bratich, however, believes that Gilbert focused on Douglass because it suited his political agenda, and that if he had looked at more "progressive" AIDS conspiracy theorists, a rather different rhetoric (and set of "articulations") could have been generated. Precisely because left-leaning thinkers are open to the idea that governments and other politically powerful agents may conspire to cause harm, Bratich suggests that AIDS conspiracy theory "might have a higher degree of articulatability to Left politics, especially in the recent age of bioterror."[24] But in suggesting possible alternative and supposedly more progressive AIDS conspiracy theorists than Douglass, Bratich comes up with two unconvincing suggestions—namely, Boyd "Ed" Graves and Leonard Horowitz.

As discussed in chapter 2, Graves and Horowitz drew on the same Soviet-Stasi misinformation as Douglass to propose a laboratory origin for AIDS. And although they are not as obviously right-wing as Douglass, neither Graves nor Horowitz are plausible progressives, or as respectable as Bratich makes them out to be.[25] Horowitz, who has been described as "the right's most visible authority on medical matters,"[26] is an acknowledged influence on Graves's work, and both Graves and Horowitz peddled unproven, alternative silver-based cures. Graves died in 2009, but Horowitz continues to employ the conspiratorial move against science as a marketing device for his range of "alternative" remedies—some of which literally defy science. For example, in marketing a product that supposedly "applies energetic vibrations for energy beings," his sales website claims that

this area of healthcare has been suppressed by the criminal drug-pushing (medical-pharmaceutical) profiteers controlling "health care" (i.e., disease control) today through their Gestapo, the FDA, and legions of Medical Manchurians—brainwashed, mind-controlled, "Medical Deities" granted licenses to kill. . . . (And they murder people all the time, and YOU KNOW THIS TO BE TRUE!). So choose a sane alternative NOW![27]

This type of conspiratorial discourse peppers the website and is easily evident to the most casual Internet surfer. The hysterical language (replete with capitals and exclamation marks) and conspiratorial moves against the establishment ought to raise a few intellectual alarm bells, yet Bratich dismisses sources listing Horowitz as a quack[28] while uncritically relying on Horowitz's own promotional material describing his enterprise as a "non profit educational corporation" and describing Horowitz's "research" into the origin of HIV as important for scientific and ethical reasons.[29] That Graves and Horowitz are depicted by Bratich as progressive alternatives to Douglass is not only ignorant about both men, but assumes that their cultropreneurial activities are irrelevant to a left-wing agenda. It also demonstrates an extraordinary suspension of judgment toward discrediting facts which ought reasonably be taken into account when assessing their credibility.

In this respect, it is not accidental that Gilbert, in his demolition of the credibility of AIDS conspiracy theories, questioned Douglass's cultropreneurial activities. He writes that Douglass "promotes a strange cure for numerous ailments—photoluminescence—in which small amounts of blood are drawn, irradiated with ultraviolet light and reinjected. . . . Treatment at his Clayton, Georgia, clinic can span several weeks and cost thousands of dollars."[30] Gilbert is obviously seeking to discredit Douglass further by pointing to these moneymaking activities and by challenging his status as a medical expert. In the conclusion to his section titled "Shyster Science," he writes: Douglass "may be an MD but he obviously has little or no background in genetics, virology, or epidemiology" and that his theories are a "bizarre cocktail of half-truths, distortions, and lies."[31] But the fact that Gilbert is making such a discrediting move is less interesting than whether there are good reasons for doing so. Whereas postmodern scholars like Bratich focus only on rhetorical strategies, the more relevant question is whether discrediting moves are justified. This, in turn, requires that we take evidence seriously and apply reason and judgment in coming to an assessment.

CREDIBILITY AND AUDIENCE

To be effective, arguments have to be well reasoned *and* speak to the interests and concerns of particular audiences. This is why Gilbert's opening discussion is about the good reasons why people may find AIDS origin conspiracy beliefs thinkable. Bogart and Thorburn similarly conclude that the "historical discrimination" which forms an important context for AIDS conspiracy beliefs has to be acknowledged if public health interventions are to gain the trust of black communities.[32] In her review of the problem posed by conspiracy beliefs for public health more broadly, Clara Rubincam also highlights the need to acknowledge historical events "that may influence suspicion or trust" as an important part of facilitating "community-owned implementation of health initiatives."[33]

Whether Gilbert was successful in changing people's minds is a moot point as no evaluation of his program was conducted and he himself attributes most behavior change to people's "personal experience with family or friends with AIDS."[34] But judging from comments posted by prisoners about Gilbert's paper, his politically sensitive approach seems to have paid off, at least for some. Consider the following response from Albert Nuh Washington, who self-identifies as a "Black Liberation Army/Black Panther Party Political Prisoner":

> David Gilbert takes us step by step to debunk false theories on the origin of AIDS. From reputable scientists we are told why these theories are invalid. But to just show that people have whack thoughts is like an insult, so David gives us very concrete reasons why Black people in particular hold such views. . . .
>
> He points us to the real genocide: disinformation and misinformation. By ignoring facts on behavior, people have left themselves open to infection—and thus in a position to infect others. The AIDS orphans of Africa bear witness to this. Ignorance is the root of all misfortune, and those who put forth these false conspiracy theories are aiding and abetting the racists who would see us destroyed.[35]

But whereas Washington was prepared to accept that truth could come from "reputable scientists," not everyone was as convinced. Another post, signed "J. Sakai" reads as follows:

> At first, like so many of us, I thought this horrifying epidemic just had to be some biological warfare experiment run loose. The often-quoted "evidence" in the writings of Dr. William Campbell Douglass, M.D., helped convince me. So it was a real eye-opener for me to learn from David Gilbert's paper that this Dr. Douglass wasn't a Black nationalist, as I'd assumed, but a white Right-wing racist whose "evidence" is all fake.
>
> To me, David Gilbert's paper is fascinating and necessary reading, but there is one side of it that I think we need to discuss more. Yes, I think his sources are right in this case. But when some scientist assures us that blah de blah is true—"Just take my word for it"—don't we all start looking for the fire escape? It's not a problem that they have sophisticated knowledge and we may not. Maybe it's precisely because the oppressed do not yet have functioning liberated sciences of our own that we have to tenaciously resist being trusting or dependent on capitalist science? I don't have a good answer for all this, but I think we have to start discussing it.[36]

Sakai's post is interesting in that it shows that, at least in this instance, Gilbert's arguments about the science of HIV and his critique of Douglass were able to have some impact on those predisposed to believing that HIV is a bioweapon. It is also interesting for the way it shows how science occupies an ambiguous position, even for those whose instincts are to distrust it. He accepts that scientists may have "sophisticated knowledge" which people lack, while articulating the need to "resist being trusting or dependent on capitalist science"—and recognizing that this is a conundrum, perhaps resolvable only under a system of socialized medicine. But that he was prepared to accept that Gilbert's sources are "right" suggests that the credibility Gilbert was able to invest in his scientist friend (from his civil rights days) and his own credibility as a revolutionary paid off in this case. It suggests that both the argument and the voice matter in challenging AIDS origin conspiracy beliefs.

5

SCIENCE, CONSPIRACY THEORY, AND THE
SOUTH AFRICAN AIDS POLICY TRAGEDY

This chapter reflects on President Mbeki's tragic questioning of HIV science and his conspiratorial move against antiretrovirals. This is an important story for two reasons. First, South Africa has more people living with HIV than any other country.[1] What happens in this middle-income developing country thus has serious implications for the global HIV epidemic. Second, it provides a clear example of the very real human consequences that can occur when leaders reject scientific expertise. It is one thing for academics to pose questions about different "ways of knowing" and about the gaps and ambiguities within scientific "facts"—but problems of an entirely different moral and social magnitude arise when policymakers adopt a form of postmodern skepticism to ignore or reject the best available evidence.

When Mbeki succeeded Mandela as president in 1999, almost one in five South African adults was already infected with HIV (see fig. 2.1). About 300,000 people had already died of AIDS, but under Mbeki's presidency the death toll skyrocketed to include another 2.7 million more. As discussed below, hundreds of thousands of these deaths could have been prevented. The South African AIDS policy debacle has been told in more detail elsewhere,[2] but the key issue was that, rather than basing AIDS policy on the scientific consensus, Mbeki took seriously the claim by self-styled "dissidents" that HIV science was fundamentally flawed and corrupted by the pharmaceutical industry. Apparently on the advice of a journalist who had sent him some of their material,[3] Mbeki convened a Presidential AIDS Advisory Panel with half the seats allocated to these critics and half to HIV scientists and clinicians. This effectively elevated a fringe set of unsupported claims to the same status as the scientific consensus on HIV pathogenesis and treatment. Commenting on the composition of the panel, John Moore, a US-based immunologist and outspoken critic of AIDS denialism, observed dryly that it comprised "pretty well everyone on it who believes that HIV is not the cause of AIDS, and about 0.0001 per cent of those who oppose this view."[4]

Meanwhile, Mbeki's health minister, Tshabalala-Msimang, rejected reports from South Africa's Medicines Control Council (MCC) that antiretrovirals were safe and effective—describing them instead as "poison."[5] As medical professionals and AIDS activists fought for an evidence-based AIDS policy, she starved the MCC of resources and obstructed donor funding for antiretrovirals. She hired Roberto Giraldo, a cultropreneur and leading member of the AIDS denialist community (see chapter 6) to promote nutritional alternatives, and she invited him to a meeting of Southern African health ministers, where he told the audience that "the transmission of AIDS from person to person is a myth" and that "malnourishment is at the centre of its progression."[6] Tshabalala-Msimang also supported other cultropreneurs in the AIDS arena, notably Mattias Rath, the vitamin magnate, who ran illegal clinical "trials" in Khayelitsha in which patients were encouraged to go off of antiretroviral treatment and onto his therapies instead—with predictably dire consequences.[7]

AIDS policy under Mbeki is particularly puzzling because the science of HIV and AIDS treatment was very well established by the time he became president in June 1999. Sixteen years earlier, Françoise Barré-Sinoussi, Luc Montagnier, and Robert Gallo had identified a retrovirus, subsequently known as HIV, as the probable cause of AIDS.[8] This was followed by rapid developments in HIV science that not only contributed significantly to virology and immunology, but made the development of antiretroviral treatment possible and increasingly effective. Inevitably, gaps in our understanding remain, particularly with regard to precisely how the immune system is destroyed and the genetic basis for why some people progress to AIDS faster than others. Even so, as a 2010 review concludes:

> Advances in understanding of HIV biology and pathogenesis, and in application of that knowledge to reduce morbidity and mortality, rank among the most impressive accomplishments in medical history. No example since penicillin rivals the development of antiretroviral drugs in controlling a previously fatal infection.[9]

The "dissidents" who caught Mbeki's attention, however, resist this conclusion by ignoring or posing questions about the evidence, contesting the validity of HIV tests, stressing the toxicity of antiretrovirals, and promoting untested alternative hypotheses. Some, like Eleni Papadopulos-Eleopulos (a medical technician at the Royal Perth Hospital in Australia) believe that HIV does not exist at all—despite the fact that HIV has been isolated and its genome fully described.[10] Others, like Peter Duesberg (a virologist at the University of California, Berkeley), believe that HIV exists, but that it is harmless and that it is antiretroviral drugs themselves that cause AIDS. As discussed in chapter 7, these claims have been countered many times by the scientific community, but for the lay person confronted by what appears to be a "genuine scientific debate" (as Mbeki apparently saw it), the matter can appear truly confusing.

One way for nonscientists (like me) to exercise some reasonable judgment on the issue is to concentrate on two undeniable and easily graspable facts—that clinical trials have shown that antiretrovirals are effective at reducing HIV transmission and extending the lives of those living with HIV; and that the scientific understanding of how antiretrovirals work is consistent with these outcomes and the basic science of HIV disease (discussed in more detail below). Given this neat dovetailing of the science of HIV pathogenesis and treatment with clinical evidence, it is reasonable to conclude that the basic science is not simply up for grabs in any fundamental sense by people proposing untested alternative hypotheses that fly in the face of the proven efficacy of antiretroviral treatment. Again, questions inevitably remain about the way that the drugs impact on the human body, but their proven efficacy at saving lives means that it is wildly disproportionate to reject the science of antiretroviral treatment because of these questions.

THE DOVETAILING OF HIV SCIENCE AND AIDS TREATMENT

There is a substantial body of evidence stretching back two decades showing that antiretroviral treatment dramatically reduces AIDS-related mortality.[11] HIV-positive people aged 20 going on antiretroviral treatment today can now expect to live into their sixties and with good quality of life.[12] By the turn of the century these dramatic effects were evident in cohort studies including patients in developing countries. Antiretroviral treatment had been shown to be possible in Haiti[13] and soon thereafter in South Africa, when Médecins Sans Frontières (MSF; aka Doctors Without Borders) demonstrated that antiretroviral treatment could restore immune function and extend life in poverty-stricken urban and rural settings.[14] When antiretroviral treatment was eventually scaled up nationally by Mbeki's successor (Jacob Zuma), the impact was evident to all, as illustrated by the gratifying headline, complete with exclamation mark in figure 5.1: "ARVs Hurt Funeral Business!"

In essence, the scientific understanding of how antiretrovirals work is that they target the known pathways of viral replication. HIV invades the immune system by attaching to CD4 molecules on the surface of T-cells (white blood cells) and entering the cell with the help of one of two coreceptors. Antiretroviral drugs known as fusion and entry inhibitors were developed precisely to block this process. Once HIV enters the cell, viral RNA (ribonucleic acid) is released along with an enzyme called reverse transcriptase, which helps turn the RNA into DNA (deoxyribonucleic acid). A further enzyme, integrase, is also released, which facilitates the integration of the new viral DNA into the T-cell's nucleus. Drugs known as reverse transcriptase inhibitors and integrase inhibitors were developed to

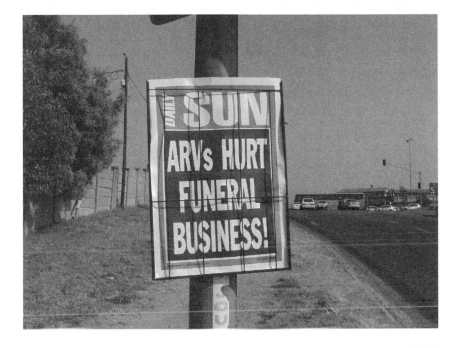

FIGURE 5.1 Headline, Johannesburg, South Africa, *Daily Sun*, October 4, 2010. (Photo courtesy of Marlise Richter)

block these processes. Finally, a further HIV enzyme, protease, assists new HIV virions (which "bud" out of the cell) develop into mature infectious particles. Protease inhibitors were developed to block this stage of HIV replication. The replication cycle is summarized in figure 5.2.

Reverse transcriptase inhibitors, notably AZT (azidothymidine), were the first antiretrovirals to be developed. While effective at lowering the viral load in pregnant HIV-positive women—thereby significantly reducing the risk of mother-to-child transmission of HIV[15]—it soon transpired that AZT was ineffective over the longer term as a monotherapy (as HIV mutated rapidly against it) and was plagued by serious side effects.[16] The key breakthrough in HIV treatment was made in the mid-1990s when scientists discovered that targeting replication at different points in the cycle made it much harder for HIV to mutate against the drug regimen.[17] The standard of care is now a triple drug "cocktail" known as highly active antiretroviral

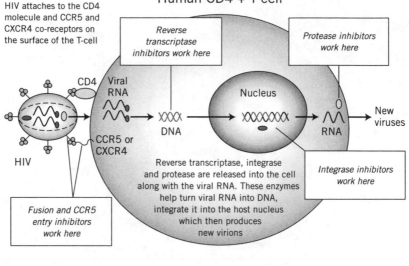

FIGURE 5.2 HIV Replication and Antiretroviral Action

treatment (HAART), which includes a protease inhibitor and at least one reverse transcriptase inhibitor.[18]

THE AIDS DENIALISTS

Yet the dissidents on Mbeki's panel remained profoundly skeptical about antiretrovirals, which is why they are commonly referred to as AIDS denialists by AIDS activists and HIV scientists. They, of course, regard the label as profoundly discrediting (which it is), seeing it as further evidence of oppression by a dominant paradigm. Dissent, of course, is central to science—but so is evidence. Genuine HIV dissidents from the 1980s who worried that there may be nonviral or cofactor causes of AIDS changed their minds once the efficacy of HAART had become apparent.[19] The label *denialist* is deserved and used unapologetically in this book. As Pride Chigwedere and others have noted, the claim that HIV causes AIDS "satisfies all three of [physician and bacteriologist Robert] Koch's postulates, the traditional standard of infectious disease causation, and all of Sir Bradford Hill's epidemiological guidelines for assessing causality."[20] To continue to assert that HIV science lacks credible evidence is simply perverse and beyond any acceptable standard of reasonable dissent.

Mbeki, however, clearly believed that scientists had not adequately considered the denialists' claims. He personally sent 1,500 pages of AIDS denialist documentation to Malagapuru Makgoba, the head of South Africa's Medical Research Council,[21] and in January 2000 he sent Makgoba and Michael Cherry (a zoologist from the University of Stellenbosch) a paper by Papadopulos-Eleopulos and others[22] arguing that because the prevailing scientific understanding of the way that AZT worked was (in her view) inadequate, whereas its toxic effects were demonstrable, the drug should not be prescribed. Mbeki sent the paper to Cherry because he had written a newspaper article quoting Makgoba as saying that he had "read nothing in the scientific or medical literature that indicates that AZT should not be provided to people."[23] Mbeki told the *Sunday Times* (South Africa):

> I wrote to the lecturer and said, "You know, it's possible that you people haven't read any such articles. Please find enclosed an article published in 1999 in a very senior scientific journal, a very lengthy article with millions of references, presenting whatever that particular group of scientists thought about that matter." There you have university people, professors and scientists who haven't read. I was very surprised in that particular incident when [Cherry] wrote back to me and said, "Mr President, I will respond to you in a fortnight, I am afraid I don't know very much about this subject. I am going to consult a friend of mine." Well, why did he write his article? What do you do if professors won't read articles about subjects they write about? What do you do?[24]

The episode is instructive on two points. First, it suggests an inability to distinguish between genuinely pathbreaking articles in top journals (like the *New England Journal of Medicine*) and the Papadopulos-Eleopulos paper, which was published by a low-ranking journal—and only in the form of a supplement which is not even posted in the journal's archive.[25] Second, it demonstrates Mbeki's disdain for Cherry's expressed need to seek advice from expert virologists and pharmacologists before responding. This suggests that Mbeki did not value the way that scientific communities exist as networks of cooperation, trust, and authority. As sociologist of science Steven Epstein puts it: "Since no one can 'know' all or even a fraction of the corpus of scientific knowledge through direct experience, science is made possible through the allocation of trust."[26] A zoologist like Cherry would thus be expected to consult with relevant experts before commenting to Mbeki on Papadopulos-Eleopulos's claims. Mbeki, however, seemed to reflect instead the common AIDS denialist stance that any determined truth seeker can come to grips with the relevant science and make an informed judgment on his or her own.

After consulting with several specialists Cherry responded to Mbeki,[27] pointing out that Papadopulos-Eleopulos had presented no original research, that her case against AZT was based on a very selective (and dated) set of references which ignored the best available science on the effectiveness of AZT, and that she had failed to weigh the problem of drug toxicity against the benefits of mother-to-child transmission prevention (MTCTP). Mbeki forwarded these comments to Papadopulos-Eleopulos, who then responded (via Mbeki) to Cherry. To every reference Cherry made to the scientific literature, she replied that none of it amounted to sufficient "proof" of the efficacy of AZT and reasserted her view that AZT could not possibly be effective while further complaining about its side effects. And, when he pointed out that one of the papers she cited in support of her argument that AZT was dangerous had concluded that AZT should be used for MTCTP, she responded by saying that the authors of that study had been forced to add that recommendation in order to have their work published.

Papadopulos-Eleopulos used a similar approach in testifying before an Australian court (in defense of Andre Parenzee, who was accused of infecting a sexual partner with HIV—see chapter 6) as to why she believed HIV does not exist. The judge ruled that she was not objective in her evidence. His comments are instructive in this regard:

She commences with a proposition which she then seeks to justify by reliance on material which, when properly understood, does not support the proposition.

Ms Papadopulos-Eleopulos propounds theories which are not supported by adequate scientific research or knowledge. She demonstrates an ability to read scientific literature but she has misused and misinterpreted much of the material upon which she seeks to rely. She takes statements out of context and then relies on them to support conclusions which are not supported by the text.

Her evidence is littered with examples of misunderstandings, misinterpretation and denial of established scientific research. In many instances she relies on material which is outdated. She either deliberately fails to acknowledge or is not aware of the most recent scientific research that establishes that HIV exists and that, if untreated, will lead to the breakdown of the immune system'.[28]

This is a succinct summary of the way in which AIDS denialists approach HIV science—and why it is impossible to engage in productive discussions with them. It is thus unsurprising that no agreement was possible between the opposing sides on Mbeki's Presidential AIDS Advisory Panel. The panel met in May 2000 and again in July that year, finally reporting in March 2001. As the final report notes: "The gallant efforts of very able facilitators did not succeed in preventing the panel from polarising into two main camps."[29] Salim Abdool-Karim presented data from King George V Hospital showing that the two-year fatality rate for children infected with HIV is almost 60 percent (22), and Makgoba provided evidence from Baragwanath Hospital that 46 out of 54 HIV-positive babies born to a cohort of HIV-positive women had died of AIDS within eighteen months and that antiretrovirals had reduced maternal transmission of HIV significantly (33). The denialists, however, disregarded such evidence and concluded that HIV testing and the use of antiretrovirals should be avoided (79, 83). David Rasnick asserted that "AIDS would disappear instantaneously" if HIV testing was outlawed and the use of antiretrovirals terminated" 15). Duesberg and Giraldo backed him up, arguing that AIDS in Africa was caused by poverty (23–24), not HIV.

By arguing that AIDS in Africa was caused by poverty and that "toxic" antiretroviral drugs were being foistered on a vulnerable population so that pharmaceutical companies could make money, the AIDS denialist argument resonated within a broader postcolonial critique of biomedicine. Indeed, humanities scholars like Didier Fassin[30] and Joy Wang[31] argue that it was this angle that especially appealed to Mbeki. They hypothesize that it was precisely because the profit-driven pharmaceutical industry neglects diseases of poverty and because Western biomedicine has been associated with social oppression—for example, slum clearances in the name of "hygiene," removals in response to smallpox, residential segregation in the name of sanitation, etc.[32]—that AIDS denialist arguments found new and fertile terrain in South Africa.

When he opened the 2000 International AIDS Conference in Durban, Mbeki infamously avoided linking HIV to AIDS while stressing the role of poverty in driving AIDS deaths in Africa.[33] While his remarks bore a close affinity to the claims of the AIDS denialists on his panel, it was not entirely unreasonable to propose a link between HIV/AIDS and poverty as there are biologically plausible pathways between poverty and HIV infection which are consistent with what has already been established about HIV pathogenesis. Precisely because HIV has to cross mucosal or skin barriers, and then find target cells to infect, relatively few people exposed to HIV through unprotected sex go on to develop an active HIV infection. It is thus possible that malnourished people are more susceptible to HIV infection if their mucosal barriers and skin integrity are accordingly compromised. Untreated ulcerative sexually transmitted infections increase the risk of HIV infection, and it is also possible that those with chronic parasitic infections will also be especially vulnerable to HIV infection as their immune systems are consequently overactivated, thus creating more target T-cells for HIV to infect.[34]

Even so, no studies have shown a clear link between HIV status and parasitic infections, and statistical analysis of potential correlates of HIV prevalence come to differing conclusions about the relative importance of poverty versus other factors.[35] This is because, in some cases, poverty has been associated with increased vulnerability to HIV (including through increased risk behaviors), whereas in other cases it is the relatively economically better off who are more vulnerable.[36] No wonder, then, that there is a lively debate about how much of the AIDS response should be targeted to "structural" (socioeconomic) factors which may underpin vulnerability to HIV infection versus explicitly biomedical and behavioral interventions. However, none of this has any bearing on the validity of HIV science or the efficacy of antiretrovirals. Thus, while it was not unreasonable for Mbeki to associate the African AIDS epidemic with poverty and to question the way in which some donors prioritize biomedical interventions over poverty and economic development, the problem was that he did this *rather than*, and *at the direct cost of*, the use of antiretrovirals for MTCTP and HAART.

In his sympathetic portrayal of Mbeki's questioning of HIV science, Fassin is critical of the "orthodoxy" for presenting state-of-the-art knowledge as definitive and indisputable and for being so "resolutely biomedical and behavioural" that room was not made for the kinds of concerns Mbeki had. Fassin, in effect, blames scientific arrogance for pushing Mbeki into the arms of the AIDS denialists.[37] While it is no doubt true that Mbeki was irritated by what he perceived to be unnecessarily definitive scientific statements, this is not a plausible justification for his conspiratorial moves against HIV science and his tragically delayed MTCTP program. A better response would have been to fund more research on poverty as a potentially neglected cause of the AIDS epidemic—while also accepting the evidence that antiretrovirals work for MTCTP and HAART. Accounts such as Fassin's, which concentrate on the "good reasons" for Mbeki's rival "logic" on AIDS while failing to critique the profoundly unreasonable and conspiratorial moves he made, are partial at best.

A similar problem besets social constructivist accounts of scientific controversies versus truth claims, and some scholars now worry that the distinction between good and bad scientific policy advice has become dangerously obscured.[38] As Harry Collins, observes, the "modern social analyst of science has no more to say about the failure of Trofim Lysenko's theories of biological inherence during Stalinist times than the failure of the Soviet Union—both simply lost a political battle."[39] He argues that policymakers need to accept scientific expertise as "real." This idea is discussed further below.

THE HUMAN COSTS OF DELAYING THE USE OF
ANTIRETROVIRALS IN SOUTH AFRICA

When Mbeki took office in 1999, clinical trials in Thailand and Uganda had shown that giving a short course of AZT or Nevirapine to HIV-positive pregnant women significantly reduced the risk of transmitting HIV to their babies—and at relatively low cost.[40] Indeed, the South African Health Ministry's Reproductive Health Director told journalists in 1998 that the success of Nevirapine trials in Uganda was "exciting news" because "there is a possibility of something fairly affordable that can be used to prevent babies being infected."[41] Pilot MTCTP sites were set up and expanded when the price of AZT (which was more efficient at MTCTP) fell by two-thirds. This initiative was later halted, initially supposedly because of affordability, but subsequently over concerns about the use of antiretrovirals themselves.[42]

In one of his first speeches as president, Mbeki raised doubts about the safety of AZT and instructed his health minister to find out "where the truth lies."[43] Two weeks later, Tshabalala-Msimang told parliament that although she was aware of positive reports about AZT (including from the MCC), there were "other scientists who say that not enough is yet known about the effects of the toxic profile of the drug, that the risks might well outweigh the benefits and that the drug should not be used."[44] She reportedly arranged a meeting between AIDS denialists and the registrar of the MCC[45] and ignored the recommendations of the World Health Organization (WHO) that AZT had an "acceptable clinical safety profile" and was an "essential drug" for MTCTP in developing countries.[46]

Mbeki and Tshabalala-Msimang were eventually forced to concede ground over MTCTP in 2002, after a court ruled in favor of a coalition of AIDS clinicians, legal activists, and the Treatment Action Campaign (TAC), and the following year the cabinet overruled Mbeki and announced that HAART would be provided through the public sector. Even so, precisely because Tshabalala-Msimang remained health minister, the use of antiretrovirals for prevention and treatment was plagued by inefficiencies and poor leadership at the national level.[47]

NOTE TO LIBRARY:

REGARDING PROCESSING

_____ CIP cataloging is only cataloging available for this title.

__✓__ There is not a MARC record available for this title.

_____ Due to the format of this book, we have not attached a polyester cover

_____ Due to the size/format of this book, we are unable to:

    _____ Supply a jacket cover.

    _____ Property stamp.

    _____ Attach a pocket/check out card/date due slip.

REGARDING BINDING

_____ The paperback cover was damaged during the binding process. Therefore, this book had to be bound in Cloth.

_____ The bindery erroneously bound this book in Vinabind instead of Cloth.

_____ Unsuitable for Vinabind. Book has been bound in Cloth.

_____ Unsuitable for binding.

_____ Perforated pages. Unsuitable for binding.

_____ Book is too thick. Unsuitable for binding.

_____ Book is too thin. Unsuitable for binding.

_____ Narrow margins. Unsuitable for binding.

_____ Fold out pages and/or covers. Unsuitable for binding.

_____ Not bound. Binding could damage attached item in book

_____ Not bound per customer request.

_____ Other:_____

MIDWEST LIBRARY SERVICE

The fact that the Western Cape Province had defied national AIDS policy by offering MTCTP services from 1999 in key hospitals, and by initiating in 2001 (in partnership with MSF) a pilot HAART project in the African township of Khayelitsha, makes the following thought experiment possible: how many HIV infections and premature deaths could have been prevented if the entire country had been encouraged to do the same? One way of answering this is to use a demographic model produced by the Actuarial Society of South Africa to estimate the impact of the HIV epidemic on the South African population.[48] This model links the increase in death rates among young adults in South Africa to rising HIV prevalence while simultaneously accounting for the positive impact of policies such as MTCTP and HAART. Users can adapt the policy assumptions of this model to run an alternative hypothetical scenario in which the Western Cape's AIDS policy stance is imagined to have been replicated nationally. Subtracting the estimated number of deaths and new infections generated by this hypothetical exercise from the totals generated by the original model (of what actually happened) thus gives an estimate of the number of deaths and new HIV infections which could have been prevented if national policy had mirrored that in the Western Cape. The results, shown in figure 5.3, indicate that about 180,000 new HIV infections and 333,000 deaths could have been prevented over the term of the Mbeki presidency. These results, an earlier version of which was published elsewhere,[49] are consistent with those of Chigwedere and others[50] using a different methodology.

Note that this estimate of unnecessary loss of life only takes into account the cost of the delayed use of antiretrovirals. It does not include the ultimately unmeasurable impact that Mbeki may have had on the demand for antiretrovirals from individuals. For example, Zambian AIDS activist Winstone Zulu described how he had been intrigued by Duesberg and his followers, but that it was when Mbeki endorsed them that he became an AIDS denialist himself. Mirroring LeRoy Whitfield's reaction to Louis Farrakhan (chapter 3), Zulu told journalist Stephanie Nolan: "Here was Thabo Mbeki, my hero—when Thabo Mbeki questioned it, I was sold."[51] Zulu subsequently resigned from his posts in various AIDS organizations and stopped taking HAART. Fortunately he came to doubt Mbeki's claim

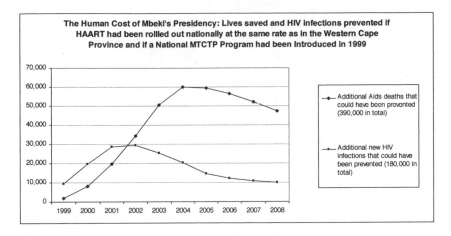

FIGURE 5.3 Estimating the Human Costs of Mbeki's AIDS Policies (using the ASSA2003 demographic model, available from http://aids.actuarialsociety.org.za/ASSA2003-Model-3165.htm).

that poverty caused AIDS because in his experience it was the better off who were hardest hit in his country. When he became sick with AIDS once more, Zulu went back on HAART and returned to AIDS activism. Commenting on his denialist phase he observed:

> What mattered to me as a person living with HIV was to be told that HIV did not cause AIDS. That was nice. Of course, it was like printing money when the economy is not doing well. Or pissing in your pants when the weather is too cold. Comforting for a while but disastrous in the long run.[52]

Zulu says he was saved by not feeling "too ashamed to go back and ask for real advice."[53] It is unknowable how many people followed Zulu's path to AIDS denialism—but without making his transition back to accepting the validity of evidence-based medicine. Well-known cases in South Africa include Peter Mokaba, a youth leader who penned an AIDS denialist piece with Mbeki and subsequently died of AIDS, and Mbeki's spokesman Parks Mankahlana, who, if he went on HAART at all, did so too late to save himself.[54] It is possible that there were many like them.

SCIENTIFIC EXPERTISE AND POLICYMAKING

That Mbeki's policies had such direct and indirect human costs raises acute questions about the role of science and scientific expertise in policymaking. Policymakers, precisely because they are taking concrete action using public resources, need to make definitive judgments about the best route to follow—even when the relevant science or knowledge base is contested, incomplete, and evolving. As sociologists of science Harry Collins and Robert Evans argue,[55] a sharp distinction should be drawn between the academic study of scientific fact-making (entailing a "symmetrical" approach to rival claims) and policymaking, which ought, in their opinion, be guided by legitimate expertise, i.e., the scientific consensus position. Although scholars working in the area of science studies have shown how rhetorical and social processes are inevitably involved in solidifying the scientific consensus position,[56] the clear implication of the Collins and Evans distinction is that policymakers should avoid becoming paralyzed or distracted by this when called upon to implement policies.

Their position, in other words, is that if Mbeki was an academic, he would have had the freedom to pose questions about the gaps in HIV science and about the processes involved in producing an overarching scientific consensus. But because he was president, he should not have abrogated himself that luxury while delaying the introduction of antiretrovirals. Those seeking to defend Mbeki on the grounds that he was merely engaging in a legitimate intellectual questioning of HIV science miss this important point.[57]

There were, in fact, some grounds for suspicion about the way that HIV science and antiretroviral treatment developed in the 1980s. Epstein documents how quickly HIV was accepted as *the* cause of AIDS even though the initial studies underpinning this conclusion framed the connection more cautiously in terms of HIV being the "probable" cause of AIDS.[58] He argues that during the mid-1980s both clinical and rhetorical factors were at work in facilitating this process of scientific fact-making and that the design and implementation of clinical trials was shaped by engagement with AIDS activists. It was thus reasonable to worry that there may have been other causes of AIDS besides HIV or that the early clinical trials of AZT were flawed. And when AZT, which initially cost over $10,000 a year and was prescribed in overly high doses,[59] eventually proved ineffective as a monotherapy, the stage was set for conspiratorial views about Big Pharma making profits out of poisonous drugs.[60]

However, with the development of more tolerable treatment regimens (especially much lower doses of AZT) and the advent of HAART, the weight of evidence and scientific and clinical opinion shifted firmly in favor of antiretrovirals. By the time that the results of the HIV Outpatients Study was published in 1998 showing the indubitable benefits of HAART,[61] most AIDS patients receiving treatment in the advanced capitalist countries were already on triple therapy.[62] AIDS denialists, however, continue to fixate on the early problems with AZT (the trial design, early problems of toxicity), effectively ignoring the subsequent development of HAART.

This obsession with AZT was evident also in South Africa. In one of the first media appearances of AIDS denialism in South Africa, Anthony Brink, a magistrate with no formal scientific training, argued that AZT was a "medicine from hell" and defended the health minister's decision not to make AZT available for MTCTP on the grounds that prescribing it "was akin to napalm-bombing a school to kill some roof-rats."[63] Des Martin, the head of the Southern African HIV Clinicians Society, responded by pointing out that antiretrovirals had resulted in a 40 percent decline in US AIDS mortality between 1995 and 1997, and that AZT has been shown to cut maternal transmission by 67 percent. He agreed that side effects are a "very real issue" requiring constant vigilance on the part of clinicians. However, its benefits for MTCTP rendered the drug in his view, "a medicine from heaven."[64] Mbeki, however, appears to have been convinced by Brink's concerns.[65]

Rather than accepting the advice of the scientific community, Mbeki set about educating himself and advised provincial leaders to access "the huge volume of literature on this matter available on the Internet."[66] In his opening address to the first meeting of his AIDS panel, Mbeki said:

> I faced this difficult problem of reading all these complicated things that
> you scientists write about, in this language I don't understand. So I ploughed

through lots and lots of documentation, with dictionaries all around me in case there were words that seemed difficult to understand. I would phone the Minister of Health and say, "Minister, what does this word mean?" And she would explain. I am somewhat embarrassed to say that I discovered that there had been a controversy around these matters for quite some time. I honestly didn't know. I was a bit comforted later when I checked with a number of our Ministers and found that they were as ignorant as I, so I wasn't quite alone.[67]

In this way, Mbeki was probably able to develop a rudimentary level of expertise. But without actually immersing himself in the scientific community (where domain-specific and tacit knowledge are to be obtained), he could never hope to achieve what Collins and Evans call the necessary "interactional" or "contributory" expertise needed to participate in the scientific community as a legitimate expert.[68] In Martin Weinel's assessment, the most Mbeki achieved was a form of "primary source knowledge" expertise,[69] i.e., insufficient for him to be formulating policy without expert input. Brink, however, disagreed. When Weinel argued on www.Politicsweb.co.za[70] that Mbeki lacked the necessary expertise to make the call on AZT, Brink wrote a rebuttal which appealed directly to the readers by asking:

> Do you agree that Mbeki should have consulted the top AIDS experts in South Africa to clue him in—all of them totally invested, personally and professionally, in the standard American approach to AIDS with AZT and similar drugs? If you do, then this might be a good time to stop reading and get on the phone to your doctor and ask him to tell you what you should think about all this, since doctor always knows what's best. Because unless you hang out at conferences and meetings and so on with the local AIDS experts . . . and you immerse yourself in their culture, their culture of indolence, ignorance, stupidity and arrogance, Mr Weinel says that you, like Mbeki, just don't have what it takes to make up your mind unassisted.'[71]

Brink is doing two things here: casting aspersions on the legitimacy of the scientific community and making a personal appeal to readers to join his brave band of free-thinking truth-seekers who refuse to believe that "doctor always knows what's best." As discussed further in chapter 6, this conspiratorial move not only enables people to deny that HIV is a problem, but provides them with a thrilling new identity of having seen the truth while boldly asserting their right to seek whatever alternative treatments they wish. Interestingly, the notion that people can find the truth through personal quest is characteristic of the cultic milieu,[72] and the arrogant claim to a special quality of character or thought required to see the truth, while casting nonbelievers as robots or "sheeple" is characteristic of conspiracy thinking in general.[73]

Brink's disdainful rejection of the legitimacy of the scientific consensus is characteristic also of the Mbeki presidency. When 5,000 scientists and physicians at the 2000 International AIDS Conference in Durban signed the "Durban Declaration"[74] that HIV caused AIDS and antiretrovirals help combat it, Mbeki's spokesman warned that if presented to Mbeki "it would find its comfortable place among the dustbins of the office."[75] The twelve AIDS denialists on Mbeki's panel also wrote a letter (published in *Nature*) rejecting the Durban Declaration,[76] which prompted a group of scientists and AIDS activists to reply by asking "why are AIDS denialists still making 15-year-old, long-refuted claims?"[77] In another letter, three vaccine researchers wrote of their concern that, "As long as Mr Mbeki is being advised by people with no credibility, we as South African scientists feel dangerously marginalised in the search for solutions to HIV/AIDS."[78]

In a televised interview Mbeki made clear his opposition to deferring to expert opinion when making policy decisions:

> I don't particularly see why health should be treated as a specialist thing and the President of a country can't take health decision [*sic*]. I think it would be a dereliction of duty if we were to say as far as health issues are concerned, we will leave it to the doctors and scientists, or as far as education is concerned, we will leave it to educationalists and pedagogues. I think that argument is absurd, actually.[79]

He made a similar point, albeit more angrily, to Tony Leon, the leader of the parliamentary opposition party, who had been calling for an MTCTP program.

The idea that as the executive, we should take decisions we can defend simply because views have been expressed by scientist-economists, scientist-agriculturalists, scientist-environmentalists, scientist-pedagogues, scientist-soldiers, scientist–health workers, scientist-communicators is absurd in the extreme. It is sad that you feel compelled to sink to such absurdity, simply to promote the sale of AZT.[80]

To suggest that those who were arguing for the use of antiretrovirals were "simply" promoting the sale of AZT is a conspiratorial move that is both discrediting and deflecting. Not only does it undermine the legitimacy of those conducting or citing the relevant science, but it implies that the evidence in favor of antiretrovirals cannot be trusted and thus in practice should be ignored. This maneuver is commonplace within the world of AIDS denialism and was clearly evident at the height of Mbeki's public questioning of HIV science.

For example, in March 2000 the Office of the President released a statement claiming that the "sole beneficiaries" of AZT were the pharmaceutical industry and the media (which obtained advertising revenues from the drug companies) and that this was "to the detriment of the millions that live with HIV and AIDS."[81] That same week, Mbeki's spokesman wrote an article in *Business Day* supporting Mbeki and harshly criticizing the pharmaceutical industry for propagating fear to increase their profits.[82] The ANC also released supportive statements calling on people to "refuse to surrender to populism, dogma and sales pitches of some pharmaceutical companies and their agents" and condemning the Khayelitsha HAART program as a "political ploy" manifesting a "total disregard for the well being and safety of our people who are being used as guinea pigs and conned into using dangerous and toxic drugs that are detrimental to their own health," claiming that it was an "onslaught directed at our people, reminiscent of the biological warfare of the Apartheid era." When Tony Leon's party (the Democratic Alliance) promised to provide MTCTP in the provincial areas it controlled, the ANC released a statement saying: "We as the ANC, warn Tony Leon to stop using our people as political guinea pigs in their endeavour to be 'get- rich-quick salespeople' for pharmaceutical companies. Our people's lives are not for sale."[83]

It is of course impossible to determine precisely what Mbeki's motivations were for resisting the scientific consensus on HIV pathogenesis and treatment. While there is a strong case that Mbeki was simply "converted" to AIDS denialism, there are a range of alternative explanations, some economic, some political.

WERE THERE ECONOMIC REASONS FOR MBEKI'S STANCE?

One possibility is that Mbeki's questioning of the science of antiretroviral treatment was a smoke screen, that the real reason was that the government believed the drugs were unaffordable and was simply reluctant to say so. The problem with this argument is that the government would have *saved* money by implementing MTCTP because the costs of treating many AIDS-sick babies would have been averted.[84] Despite internal government documents pointing this out,[85] Mbeki's government resisted MTCTP, opting instead to fight a legal challenge from TAC and its allies all the way to the Constitutional Court, South Africa's highest court.

But what about HAART? Treating AIDS patients for life is a much more daunting economic proposition than MTCTP. However, by the time that TAC won its legal battle over MTCTP in 2002 and started to push for a HAART rollout, generic formulations and competition had reduced drug prices to much more manageable proportions. Nathan Geffen (the TAC's research head) and I calculated in early 2003 that a HAART rollout was economically feasible in South Africa, although some increase in tax revenue was probably needed.[86] Yet it took a cabinet revolt against Mbeki and Tshabalala-Msimang to achieve government commitment to rolling out HAART. Even so, and despite further sharp declines in antiretroviral prices and growing evidence of the cost-effectiveness of providing HAART,[87] the rollout proceeded at a disappointingly slow pace. It was only once Mbeki was deposed as president and after Tshabalala-Msimang died that real energy and commitment was injected into South Africa's HAART rollout.

The story, in short, suggests that the Mbeki government actively resisted MTCTP and HAART, even though both were affordable (and even cost-saving). Some scholars nevertheless suspect that the scale of the necessary response and concern about institutional capacity may well have been a factor predisposing the government to "delay and obfuscation."[88] After all, with South Africa topping the international charts in terms of the number of people needing HAART, it is possible that Mbeki believed the government lacked the necessary capacity to implement a rollout. However, given that other developing countries at lower levels of development were able to achieve higher levels of HAART coverage than South Africa, this "resource constraint" argument should not be accepted too quickly. Statistical analysis of the determinants of HAART coverage internationally suggests that after taking into account the size and distribution of the HIV-positive population, state capacity, the reach of the health sector, donor funding, per capita income, and so on, South Africa performed significantly below "expected" levels.[89] In other words, judging by international standards and taking into account South Africa's resources and demographic challenges, a far higher level of HAART coverage should have been possible.

Another proposed economic rationale for South Africa's AIDS policies is more venal and conspiratorial. Could the national government have been resisting antiretrovirals because the ANC had a stake in the development of a rival remedy? Political analyst James Myburgh insinuates as much in his account of the "Virodene" saga.[90] This scandal first came to public attention in 1997 when University of Pretoria scientists, Ziggie and Olga Visser, claimed that dimethylformamide, an industrial solvent they called "Virodene," appeared to help AIDS patients, but that their attempts to test the cure were being blocked by the "AIDS establishment." In an unprecedented move, the Vissers were invited to a cabinet meeting with some of their patients. Writing in the ANC magazine, *Mayibuye*, Mbeki described what a "privilege" it was "to hear the moving testimonies of AIDS sufferers who had been treated with Virodene, with seemingly very encouraging results."[91] The cabinet then resolved to help the Vissers win approval (from the MCC) for a scientific drug trial, and it was subsequently revealed that the ANC also provided funding and obtained a 6 percent stake in their business.[92]

In this respect, there are distinct echoes with the Kenyan experience, where on the basis of initial trials of Kemron (chapter 3) President Daniel arap Moi threw his weight behind this supposed miracle AIDS cure.[93] After this particular dream disintegrated, one of the scientists involved, Arthur Obel, developed another AIDS cure which he called "Pearl Omega." Despite the Kenyan health minister's dismissing it as a "herbal concoction," Obel managed to win the support of Moi for this drug too, apparently by arguing that the scientific community was against him and comparing himself to "historical figures who made important discoveries that were initially treated with scepticism."[94] Media coverage of Kemron and Pearl Omega was subsequently linked to declining condom use and rising HIV incidence amongst sex workers in Nairobi.[95]

Mbeki appears to have been similarly embroiled in the development of alternative remedies to antiretrovirals, but unlike Moi, he did this well after HAART had been shown to be effective. And unlike Kemron, which was tested in Kenya and the United States, the South African regulatory authorities never allowed clinical trials of Virodene. The drug was eventually tested on Tanzanian soldiers, apparently with financial support channeled through the ANC and ANC-aligned businessmen, and found to be ineffective.[96] In Myburgh's rather cynical take on the story, it was the failure of the Tanzanian trials that marked the true turning point in the ANC's approach to antiretrovirals. But the fact that Mbeki continued to hold AIDS denialist beliefs long after that points to a more deep-seated suspicion of the science of antiretrovirals on his part. This, in turn, suggests that the key reason for South Africa's misguided AIDS policy was rooted in Mbeki's "AIDS denialism."

THE ENIGMA OF MBEKI'S QUESTIONING OF HIV SCIENCE

In practice, Mbeki was not merely "questioning" HIV science or simply attempting to foster debate: he was actively choosing sides by preventing the introduction of proven lifesaving drugs into a country in the grip of a rampant AIDS epidemic. And although he never publicly stated that

HIV does not cause AIDS, he never said it did either, thereby not only denying the government's HIV-prevention program any high-level support, but actively sowing confusion about the need for HIV testing, MTCTP, or HAART. Even after he announced his "withdrawal" from public commentary on HIV science in October 2000, he continued to dispute death statistics attributed to AIDS and, when asked on television in April 2001 if he would take an HIV test, he refused on the grounds that it would be "setting an example within the context of a particular paradigm."[97] He also probably coauthored an AIDS denialist tract with Peter Mokaba,[98] an updated version of which he sent to Mark Gevisser, who was writing Mbeki's biography at the time. For Gevisser, the message Mbeki was delivering was clear: "he was now, as he had been since 1999, an AIDS dissident."[99]

Why did Mbeki question HIV science—even to the point of harming himself politically? Some argue that the saga is best understood as part of a political struggle with civil society. Thus once he encountered resistance from scientists, AIDS activists, and health professionals—all of whom could mobilize different forms of social and political capital—he was locked into a battle over the nature of state power itself.[100] But this begs the question why he put himself in the position of having to struggle against mainstream opinion on AIDS in the first place.

Another interpretation, also focusing on political determinants, emphasizes Mbeki's revolutionary political socialization, which may have predisposed him to seeing science as corrupted by industrial interests.[101] Even so, none of this explains why Mbeki fought the battle so hard, and at such political cost, or why his supposedly revolutionary AIDS policy was so out of step with his own support for the government's orthodox economic policies. Gevisser suggests that Mbeki's appropriation of a radical critique of Big Pharma may have been an attempt to find a home for his left-wing heritage that had been lost through his orthodox stance on economics,[102] but while intriguing, this remains speculative.

A different set of explanations for Mbeki's position on AIDS highlights his anticolonial, Africanist ideology and especially his desire not to see Africa "blamed" for a sexually driven epidemic.[103] That Mbeki aligned himself with this view is incontrovertible. In an infamous public lecture in October 2001, he proclaimed:

> And thus does it happen that others who consider themselves to be our
> leaders take to the streets carrying their placards, to demand that because
> we are germ carriers and human beings of a lower order that cannot subject
> its passions to reason, we must perforce adopt strange opinions, to save a
> depraved and diseased people from perishing from self-inflicted disease.[104]

This statement is almost certainly a reference to the TAC—the "others"
who, by virtue of demanding access to AIDS treatment, were supposedly
endorsing a derogatory view of African sexuality (presumably because
TAC accepts that HIV is sexually transmitted) and trying to force government to adopt "strange opinions" (that is, to accept that antiretrovirals
save lives). And the paper he probably coauthored with Mokaba, entitled
"Castro Hlongwane, Caravans, Cats, Geese, Foot and Mouth Statistics:
HIV/AIDS and the Struggle for the Humanisation of the African," angrily condemns Western negative stereotypes about African sexuality.[105]
This document, as Joy Wang points out, is framed in a postcolonialist discourse in which acceptance of antiretrovirals is portrayed as tantamount to
humiliating subjugation to the West. She highlights the references in the
document to Fanon and hypothesizes that it was "the ANC's acceptance of
Fanon's critique of Western medicine that is at the root of the resistance to
antiretrovirals."[106]

Yet the paper relies far more on the work of AIDS denialists from the advanced capitalist countries (notably Duesberg, Giraldo, and Papadopulos-
Eleopulos) than it does on Fanon. Furthermore, it is Herbert Marcuse's
reading of social structures of power and influence as an "omnipotent apparatus" subjecting nonconformity to ridicule and defeat[107] that occupies
the conceptual center stage. The paper depicts the omnipotent apparatus as
a real conspiratorial object:

> in the name of science and friendship with the Africans, the omnipotent
> apparatus of which Marcuse wrote, has sought to present honest questions
> as a manifestation of unacceptable non-conformity. It has done everything
> it could and continues to act, to punish those who dare to ask questions. It
> uses its might, sustained by the self-repression of the African, to ensure the
> permanent repression of those who inquire.[108]

The reader is told that the omnipotent apparatus "disapproves" of the effort to deal with health, poverty, and underdevelopment and "is determined that it will stop at nothing until its objectives are achieved."[109] The fight against it is accordingly cast in bold adversarial terms, with readers warned that "we have to accept that the search for the truth will be denounced and punished by the omnipotent apparatus as unacceptable non-conformity."[110] The paper is noteworthy also for the way that scientists (derided as "geese") are seen as part of the omnipotent apparatus whereas those who support science are scorned as "cats" befriending elephants.[111]

In other words, to read this paper as a piece of anticolonial writing misses the fact that it mirrors the standard self-aggrandizing rhetoric so essential to AIDS denialism and AIDS conspiracy writing. It is far more than mere Africanism—it is part of a global conspiracist genre built on the twin pillars of a conspiratorial move against science coupled with a narcissistic portrayal of the author and his followers as the truly enlightened.

Several scholars have linked Mbeki's suspicion of medical science to its oppressive use by colonial powers, the idea being that Mbeki was speaking to this history and its supposed ongoing resonance in society.[112] But these speculations are not based on any systematic evidence about how widespread these beliefs actually are, and they fly in the face of evidence to the contrary. As historian Howard Phillips notes, by the time the AIDS epidemic appeared, biomedicine had thoroughly permeated South African society.[113] Furthermore, the fact that the TAC was able to garner significant support, including from the predominantly African trade unions, speaks to a strong social current of trust in scientific medicine within South African society. As the health and safety coordinator of the National Council of Unions put it, "we in the unions pledge our support to the roll-out of scientifically proven medication where and when necessary and we oppose those who peddle untested nostrums on a pseudo scientific basis."[114] Statements such as these suggest that it is a mistake to link Africanism with an anti–medical science perspective. Furthermore, the fact that Mbeki's very traditionalist successor, Jacob Zuma, took a strong stand against AIDS denialism and energized the HAART rollout soon after becoming president also speaks to the limitations of these ethnographic musings about how representative Mbeki's views actually were.

Consider these pained reflections by Lionel Mtshali, the premier of KwaZulu Natal Province, when he announced in February 2002 that he could no longer abide by the national government's stance on Nevirapine:

> We shall not wait one day longer, nor allow any space for further excuse, delaying tactic or preposterous theory which may get in the way of saving our children. . . . For me this is a matter of principle and common decency. I have turned upside-down the scientific facts to find a reason which can justify the failure to act and ameliorate the suffering and reduce the death of so many of our children, [and] I have found none. The undisputed facts before me are that there are sound scientific bases on which Nevirapine is recommended, which include that it is effective in reducing the number of HIV/AIDS infected babies born to HIV-positive mothers. It is cost-effective in that it is more expensive not to treat and it is safe. There to me is where the issue stops.[115]

Those who construe Mbeki's thinking on AIDS as reflecting "the reality of politics in his country"[116] cannot account for Mbeki's isolation on this issue within his own party. For example, in 2001, following public hearings on the impact of AIDS on women, a parliamentary report adopted an explicitly scientific approach and concluded that women had a right to MTCTP.[117] Similarly, at an ANC National Executive Council meeting, the ANC's National Health Secretary, Saadiq Kariem, responded furiously to the "Castro Hlwongane" paper, saying, "Anyone who believes the claims made in it might as well believe the moon is made of green cheese."[118] Finally, it is interesting that internal accounts of Mbeki's influence over AIDS policy in the early 2000s account are framed not in terms of his playing to racial fears and constructions around sexuality and HIV, but rather in organizational terms—as the ANC being paralyzed by misplaced confidence in Mbeki's intellect, loyalty to the leader, and fear of speaking out against the president.[119] If anything, it was Mbeki's leadership that caused, rather than reflected some underlying source of, the problem.

Ultimately, the reason why Mbeki championed the cause of AIDS denialism is probably relatively simple and highly personal: that AIDS denialism resonated with him intellectually; and then, for reasons relating to his personality, he refused to concede ground. As AIDS activist Zackie Achmat sees it, "He is like Macbeth. . . . It's easier to walk through the blood than to turn back and admit you made a mistake."[120] William Gumede, who penned the first biography of Mbeki, similarly points to Mbeki's stubborn arrogance, noting that he "stoically believes that he is a modern-day Copernicus who will ultimately be vindicated, even if posthumously."[121] Gevisser, in a later biography, made the same point, but located it in a wider context:

> Thabo Mbeki is a prophet-in-the-wilderness. This is what gets him up in the morning. This is what gets him through the day. He was the one who said, when nobody else believed it, that the ANC had to embrace the market and the West if it was to survive. He was deeply unpopular for it, but he was proven right. He was the one who said, at the height of the conflict, "Lay down your guns and talk to the enemy." He was called a traitor . . . a black Englishman in tweeds. But he was right, again. Now, in the era of the dream deferred, in the difficult transition, he found himself once more in a tiny minority of free-thinking dissidents. Once more, he might by overwhelmed by conventional thinking. But once more, in the long run—he believes, with absolute conviction—he will be proven correct.[122]

Gevisser's comment is insightful not only about Mbeki's personality but in pointing to the allure of being part of a "tiny minority of free-thinking dissidents." AIDS denialism is not simply about intellectual beliefs, it is about identity—and a very specific identity at that, namely as self-aggrandizing "free-thinker," or as Gumede puts it, as a modern day Copernicus. But interestingly, despite the egoistical bent to this identity, it is very much also a group or social identity. Becoming an AIDS denialist is not simply a matter of intellectual conversion, it is also about becoming a member of a group defined primarily in opposition to the science of AIDS. It is to a discussion of this community that we now turn.

6

HERO SCIENTISTS, CULTROPRENEURS, LIVING ICONS, AND PRAISE-SINGERS

AIDS DENIALISM AS COMMUNITY

Chapter 5 argues that South Africa's AIDS policy tragedy is rooted in Mbeki's involvement with AIDS denialism. It is unclear to what extent he embraced this position as his stance was typically a "questioning,"[1] one couched in a discourse of seeking to promote scientific debate in order to discover the "truth." But in so doing, he mirrored three key characteristics of AIDS denialism: extreme skepticism toward the science of HIV pathogenesis and treatment; ignoring advances in antiretroviral treatment; and the active promotion of alternative, unproven therapies in its place.

Mbeki and Tshabalala-Msimang appear to have been open to a range of counter-narratives about AIDS, some of them mutually contradictory: Mbeki articulated conspiracy theories about the pharmaceutical industry and the CIA's involvement in HIV science while also entertaining the notion that HIV was either harmless (Peter Duesberg) or that it did not even exist (Eleni Papadopulos-Eleopulos); and Tshabalala-Msimang circulated William Cooper's claims that HIV was a bioweapon, but also hired Roberto Giraldo, who denies that HIV is a pathogen, to promote nutritional solutions to immunodeficiency. But the common thread underpinning these diverse propositions is a fundamental distrust of HIV science and AIDS treatment and support for unproven alternative remedies.

Mbeki and Tshabalala-Msimang, however, did more than *entertain* counter-establishment possibilities: they *acted* on them. Whether they really believed that HIV could be a bioweapon or that it might not even exist is of limited practical relevance. The fact that they believed that the science of antiretrovirals was sufficiently problematic that they were prepared to gamble the lives of South African citizens by promoting untested alternatives means that they *de facto* made a conspiratorial move against HIV science by assuming that it was fundamentally flawed.

The idea, common in the cultic milieu, that medical science has entirely lost its way and that we are better off experimenting with alternative healing modalities is a persistent theme within organized AIDS denialism. Christine Maggiore, the deceased HIV-positive founder of the organization Alive and Well, argued that HIV-positive people must liberate themselves from "unfounded fear," avoid "toxic" antiretrovirals, and embrace their "natural ability to be well."[2] Similarly, Duesberg, along with the other AIDS denialists on Mbeki's panel, recommended that HIV testing be stopped because it was causing harmful panic and that immune deficiency be treated with nutritional interventions including herbs and garlic, "complementary" or "indigenous" remedies, and "detoxification" therapy including "massage therapy, music therapy, yoga, spiritual care, homeopathy, Indian Ayurvedic medicine, light therapy and many other methods."[3]

Such eclectic favoring of anything-other-than-medical-science is a defining feature of what may loosely be termed the "AIDS denialist community." Jeremy Youde argues that this like-minded group of people comprises a "counter epistemic community."[4] An alternative way of thinking about it is to conceive of AIDS denialism as part of the "oppositional counterculture" that emerged as part of the cultic milieu in the 1960s and then widened in scope through the incorporation of new social movements (e.g., anti-globalization)[5] and growing demand for alternative medicine.

Some of today's alternative remedies and practices originated in Europe (e.g., homeopathy, chiropractic) and others from the Orient (e.g., Ayurvedic medicine, Shiatsu, traditional Chinese medicine)—and yet others draw on an eclectic range of mystical influences and pure invention from within the cultic milieu. Common to all is that they rest on biomedically implausible mechanisms and rely on the placebo effect for their efficacy.[6] Many have been tested in clinical trials and proven ineffective,[7] but other preparations and practices are impossible to evaluate as they are geared specifically to individual clients.[8] Yet demand for them appears to have grown steadily, especially over the past couple of decades.[9]

This has been attributed to the rise of "New Age" ideas, values, and practices in which modern drugs are looked on suspiciously as "chemical," "toxic," and "unnatural," and science and technology increasingly viewed as harmful for people.[10] According to a survey in the United States, users of alternative medicine do so primarily because they find these health care choices to be "congruent with their own values, beliefs, and philosophical orientations towards health and life."[11] The notion, previously a characteristic of the cultic milieu, that patients can find their "own truths" by exploring a range of healing modalities has entered the mainstream. This, and related suspicion of science and technology, was by the end of the twentieth century already encouraging the rejection of doctors as authoritative in favor of patients themselves controlling the process of healing.[12]

Susan Harding and Kathleen Stewart argue that this new "therapeutic culture" is rooted in postmodern anxieties about the capitalist order and loss of individual agency. They argue that the link between it and tolerance for conspiracy theory is not accidental in that

> both claim a sublime pleasure in revealed knowledge and hermeneutic mastery, in the effort to uncover and recover lost or secreted knowledge, cracking codes, sifting through signs, symptoms and over-determined webs of feeling in search of the telling detail. . . . Both uncover an underlying plot that combines radical doubt with the sense that the truth is out there.[13]

But while AIDS denialists and their associated cultropreneurs clearly fit within this broader therapeutic culture, AIDS denialism is more socially substantive than this. Just as norms and values within the "scientific community" make collaboration and progress possible (discussed further in chapter 7), the AIDS denialist community has a social life which underpins the persistence and propagation of its core ideas. When Mbeki surfed the

Internet, he did not simply come across "ideas"—he would have encountered an organized network of activists who, through their linked websites, conferences, papers, books, documentaries, and public relations exercises, construct not only a rival ideology to science, but an alternative social world with its own heroes, values, beliefs, and practices. Someone doing this today encounters an even richer vein of electronic resources and connections including Facebook, video postings on YouTube, discussion groups, and blog postings. This has facilitated the growth of cyber-communities within the cultic milieu, or even, as David Aaronovitch evocatively puts it, "shadow armies whose size and power is unknowable."[14]

It is the combination of the message and the organized efforts to promote it that makes AIDS denialism such a problem for HIV scientists and activists. As the founder of *AIDS Treatment News* John James observes:

> The denialists regularly deny that precautions against infection are necessary, deny that HIV testing is appropriate, deny that any approved treatments should be used (or CD4 or viral load tests to monitor disease progression), deny that treatment saves lives, and often deny that AIDS is a real epidemic, or even a real medical condition. The problem is not ideas, but the organized efforts to practice bizarre medicine, telling people with a major illness to reject care entirely.[15]

Figure 6.1 shows the organizational connections between key AIDS denialists, including those who served on Mbeki's panel and signed the letter to *Nature* rejecting the Durban Declaration.[16] Many are active in AIDS denialist groups, organizing and attending occasional conferences, and serving on the boards of Rethinking AIDS[17] and Alive and Well. Most also featured in Brent Leung's 2009 film *House of Numbers*, to date the most prominent AIDS denialist "documentary." There are many other AIDS denialists, but this particular group is notable for its activism and role in community-building.

There are many reasons why people may be attracted to AIDS denialism: it reinforces the normal psychological processes of denial that people experience when diagnosed with a dread disease;[18] it accords with a prior distrust of medical science and the pharmaceutical industry (thereby

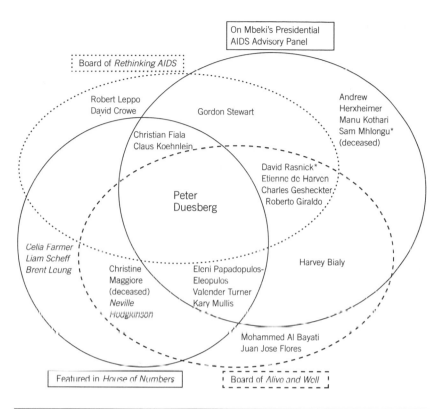

FIGURE 6.1 AIDS denialist networks: some key players (names in italics are journalists).

*Also linked to Mattias Rath

Invited onto Mbeki's panel but did not attend.

appealing to those already attracted by the cultic milieu); and it is attractive to the suspiciously minded and to those who enjoy the self-image of bold seeker challenging the orthodoxy. Buying into the world of AIDS denialism is seemingly empowering and exciting; one has joined an elect few and is bravely speaking truth to power and pushing the frontiers of genuine science, liberty, and freedom. These psychological benefits play out socially in the shared conviction that "we" are being persecuted, attacked, and bullied by a hostile, venal, and untrustworthy scientific establishment.

But while these psychological dynamics drive AIDS denialism for individuals, the AIDS denialist community is reinforced, if not made possible by, four organizationally and symbolically important roles: hero scientist, cultropreneur, living icon, and praise-singer. The hero scientist legitimates the rejection of mainstream science; the cultropreneur holds out the promise of alternative cures; and the living icon provides living proof of the concept. Praise-singers (i.e., sympathetic journalists and filmmakers) broadcast the message of the movement to the public. But precisely because these roles are important, they also provide clear targets for those seeking to combat AIDS denialism. HIV scientists have challenged the "hero scientist" on many occasions, and anti-denialist websites and blogging activities highlight the biases of the praise-singers, report the deaths of living icons, and expose the material interests and unsubstantiated and false claims of the cultropreneurs.

THE HERO SCIENTIST AS SOURCE OF CREDIBILITY AND LEGITIMACY

AIDS denialism has more credibility than AIDS origin conspiracy theories because credentialed scientists are involved. As the Zambian AIDS activist Winstone Zulu noted, when reflecting on his period of AIDS denialism, it was the "impressive scientific and medical backgrounds" of key players like Duesberg, Kary Mullis, and David Rasnick that made it difficult for him to "tell who was really in the know" about HIV and AIDS treatment.[19] Duesberg is the central "hero scientist" because he actively promotes his views to the public and has scientific qualifications that lend his views credibility.

As his supporters routinely point out, Duesberg was elected to the National Academy of Sciences in 1986 and awarded the honor of an Outstanding Investigator Research Grant from the National Institutes of Health (NIH) for his early work on viral causes of cancer. But he changed direction in the mid-1980s to claim that all retroviruses including HIV are harmless, that AIDS is not an infectious disease, and that immunodeficiency is caused by malnutrition (among poor people and those addicted to narcotics) and by recreational drugs ("mainly the ones that are used by the gays" and, "especially, AZT itself").[20] He applied to the NIH for funding to support these claims, but was unsuccessful and now relies on private donors such as Robert Leppo (on the board of Rethinking AIDS, discussed further below).

Duesberg and his supporters attribute his failure to obtain NIH funding to unfair oppression by a threatened scientific establishment.[21] His critics, however, stress that Duesberg's claims and hypotheses simply were not strong enough to succeed in the competitive world of NIH-funded research and that his initial questioning of the relationship between HIV and AIDS had hardened, without any evidence, into unsupported and unreasonable claims that HIV does not cause AIDS.[22]

Duesberg certainly has scientific credentials, but not in HIV research, and in making these claims HIV scientists regard him as commenting on an area of science he knows very little about—i.e., as lacking the necessary constitutive expertise in that field. As Robert Gallo said in an interview, he would never argue with Duesberg about "the electron spin resonance in a molecule of organic compound" (about which Duesberg has expertise)—but that, conversely, when it came to AIDS, Duesberg was totally out of his depth: "Peter doesn't understand the biology of what he is talking about. . . . He doesn't know what it means to prove something causes something or to demonstrate it . . . [and] he knows less than most people about the biology of the system, medicine and about epidemiology."[23]

The clash between AIDS denialists and HIV scientists is far more than a clash between two groups of "highly credentialed experts," as suggested by Youde.[24] It is a clash between a very large group of experts in HIV science and medicine and a small group of critics who have strong views but no relevant expertise in the fields of HIV clinical or laboratory research, or AIDS epidemiology. In short, they lack the necessary expertise to make legitimate scientific contributions in these fields. Yet this has not prevented them from dismissing the science of HIV as fraudulent, making strong claims about the number of AIDS deaths and epidemiology of AIDS in Africa (see chapter 7) and risking the lives of others through their erroneous policy advice.

It is this potential to do harm that most upsets HIV scientists and clinicians. Mark Wainberg, a Canadian microbiologist and former president of the International AIDS Society, expressed his moral outrage with Duesberg on this issue, calling him "probably the closest thing we have in this world to a scientific psychopath."[25] Duesberg's supporters, however, interpret and deflect such remarks as evidence of a conspiracy against him.[26] According to Celia Farber, an independent journalist and Duesberg's leading praise-singer, "As AIDS grew in the 1980s into a global, multibillion-dollar juggernaut of diagnostics, drugs, and activist organizations, whose sole target in the fight against AIDS was HIV, condemning Duesberg became part of the moral crusade."[27]

Seth Kalichman, a psychologist and editor of *AIDS and Behavior*, suggests in his book *Denying AIDS* that Duesberg's competitive relationship with Robert Gallo—and the much publicized and politicized dispute over whether Gallo's lab or the Pasteur Institute (Luc Montagnier and Françoise Barré-Sinoussi) discovered HIV[28]—are important contexts for AIDS denialism. Certainly, as sociologist Steven Epstein has pointed out, "the cloud of suspicion that hung over Gallo following his dispute with Luc Montagnier cast doubt on any and all claims he put forward, while Duesberg seemed credible precisely because he was challenging an entrenched and untrustworthy orthodoxy."[29] Suspicions were raised in the media[30] about whether Gallo "stole" the French virus, a problem that was ultimately traced in a subsequent investigation to widespread contamination of viral samples used in several laboratories, including Gallo's and Montagnier's,[31] and about the scientific claims Gallo made in his early publications. An exhaustive investigation eventually cleared Gallo of any misconduct, yet AIDS denialists—like the AIDS origin conspiracy theorists—obsessively and unfairly paint him as the archetypal evil figure in the great "HIV lie." As recently as December 2008, AIDS denialists wrote, unsuccessfully, to *Science* to demand the retraction of all the papers published in 1984 by Gallo's lab—supposedly because they all "relied" on questionable photographic evidence.[32] Such fixation on Gallo's early contributions reflects the common denialist trope that HIV science rests on a rotten foundation which, if exposed, will bring the entire edifice tumbling down.

This, of course, is also intellectually and organizationally convenient because it legitimates a focus on the early days of AIDS science—i.e., at the point AIDS denialists believe the scientific project went off track—and excuses them from taking seriously subsequent research reinforcing the link between HIV and AIDS and the efficacy of antiretrovirals. Mbeki himself clearly bought the claim that HIV science lost its moorings in 1984. In a letter to world leaders in April 2000 he specifically complained about "scientists in the name of science . . . demanding that we should cooperate with them to freeze scientific discourse on HIV/AIDS at the specific point this discourse had reached in the West in 1984."[33]

David Rasnick—who has coauthored papers with Duesberg and, most infamously, was associated with Mattias Rath's Khayelitsha "trials" in which South Africa AIDS patients were illegally taken off antiretrovirals and put onto the Rath Health Foundation's vitamin products instead (and with tragic consequences)[34]—is another pretender to the role of hero scientist. The Alive and Well website claims he is the "creator" of protease inhibitors. However, his name does not appear on any of the relevant patents, and his research record is notable primarily for its coauthored papers with Duesberg. As Duesberg's biographer observes, Rasnick has been important in helping to keep Duesberg's ideas in the public sphere.[35]

Another oft-cited "hero scientist" for the AIDS denialist community is Kary Mullis, an eccentric chemist who won the Nobel Prize for inventing the polymerase chain reaction, one of the technologies used for measuring HIV viral load. Mullis, who openly discusses his experimentation with hallucinatory drugs and alleged encounters with extraterrestrials, is also skeptical about HIV science,[36] despite never having done any scientific research on HIV. He has endorsed the writings of Duesberg, but is not particularly active or engaged in AIDS denialism. His disinterest and incoherence on the subject is evident in the following interview (on his website) when he said in response to a question about AIDS: "the AIDS scientists say you can cure HIV if you want to, but you still don't cure AIDS, because the disease has already done something to you. In terms of an infectious disease it's kind of an oddball thing. I don't think most of the research is reliable and I am not willing to spend a lot of effort on it."[37] However, precisely because he won a Nobel Prize, the AIDS denialist community promotes him as one of their hero scientists.

Duesberg and his support-base in Rethinking AIDS have been challenged by a rival organization, the "Perth Group,"[38] headed by Eleni Papadopulos-Eleopulos (see chapter 5). This group claims that HIV does not even exist, and once offered a reward for anyone who could prove that it did. When Duesberg sent in an entry (saying HIV did exist but was harmless), the Perth Group rejected it as not providing sufficient "evidence" for them[39] (a rather amusing episode demonstrating the difficulties of resolving disputes with AIDS denialists—even when united against the scientific orthodoxy). The division between the Perth Group and Rethinking AIDS has become sharper since members of these two groups crossed swords in Mbeki's Presidential AIDS Advisory Panel over what sorts of experiments should be conducted on HIV tests and later on how best to testify in an Australian court in the case of Andre Parenzee.

Andre Parenzee was accused of endangering human life by misleading his sexual partners about his HIV-positive status (and infecting one of them with HIV). The trial was potentially important for organized AIDS denialism because it provided a new forum—the legal system—for challenging the authority of HIV science. There have been several other attempts (in the United States) to use the legal system to rule against HIV science and antiretrovirals, but these were thrown out of court in the early stages of the proceedings.[40] With the Parenzee trial, a new opportunity arose to challenge HIV science in the public sphere—especially given that Gallo was testifying for the prosecution.[41] Unfortunately for the Rethinking AIDS group, Parenzee's defense called Papadopulos-Eleopulos and Valendar Turner (an emergency room physician and cofounder of the Perth Group) as expert witnesses rather than Duesberg or any of his supporters.

The outcome was embarrassing for the Perth Group. In his affidavit,[42] Turner testified that HIV had never been isolated (and thus could not be said to exist) because it had been identified only through the detection of reverse *transcription*—i.e., the process of writing RNA into DNA which is not unique to retroviruses. In subsequent testimony for the prosecution, Gallo[43] pointed out that HIV had actually been identified as a retrovirus through the detection of reverse *transcriptase*, which is an enzyme unique to retroviruses, not the more general activity of reverse transcription *per se*. He added that "only a fool" would mistake the two. The judge ruled that neither Turner nor Papadopulos-Eleopulos[44] had any relevant expertise and hence that their "opinion evidence" was inadmissible.[45] Rethinking AIDS then blamed the Perth Group for the disaster, saying that Duesberg would have been a more credible witness, and the Perth Group blamed Rethinking AIDS for contacting (and they claim confusing) the defense lawyer late in the trial—prompting an amused anti–AIDS denialist blogger known as "Snout" to call the AIDS denialist community a "seriously dysfunctional family."[46]

Duesberg and his organization Rethinking AIDS are fortunate in being supported by Robert Leppo, who funds some if not all of Duesberg's research and sits on the board of Rethinking AIDS. According to Farber, Leppo has funded many of their actions, including a "blitzkrieg" on Capitol Hill in 1999 in which every member of Congress received a copy of Duesberg's book *Inventing the AIDS Virus* and an excerpt from Mullis's biography.[47] Farber describes Leppo as the "reluctant hero of the underground," who by that stage had contributed more than a million dollars to the "dissident cause" and had "saved Duesberg from utter dissolution after the NIH severed his federal funding as punishment for advancing a scientific hypothesis that differed from that of the establishment."[48]

Leppo was also the "executive producer" of an AIDS denialist film, *The Other Side of AIDS* (2004), made by Robin Scovill, Maggiore's husband. The promotional material describes Leppo as a venture capitalist with an "abiding interest in Libertarian philosophy" who is also "deeply involved in researching new medical protocols and alternative therapies, many of which are AIDS related."[49] Whether his interest in AIDS denialism is purely philosophical or also material is unknown. But the connection between AIDS denialism and the marketing of alternative therapies is evident with regard to the cultropreneurs who form a further pillar for the AIDS denialist movement.

CULTROPRENEURS AND THE PROMISE OF A CURE

Earlier chapters have shown that the twinning of the conspiratorial move against science with the promotion of alternative cures is common among those promoting AIDS origin conspiracy beliefs—notably the cultropreneurs Leonard Horowitz (who sells Tetrasilver), Louis Farrakhan (who promoted Kemron), and Boyd Graves (Tetrasil). The same twinning is evident in the AIDS denialist community, even though, as Tara Smith and Steven Novella point out, this results in an internal inconsistency within AIDS denialism in that it dismisses HIV science as biased by drug money while uncritically accepting "the testimony of HIV deniers who have a heavy financial stake in their alternative treatment modalities."[50]

When the hero scientists claim that antiretrovirals are toxic and HIV science cannot be trusted, they create the perfect opening for alternative healers of all descriptions to offer solutions for staying well. These include Mattias Rath, whose Rath Health Foundation claims its multivitamins "reverse the course of AIDS"[51] and that antiretrovirals are a form of genocide inflicted on society by the "pharmaceutical drug cartel,"[52] and Gary Null, who produces audio and video posts featuring AIDS denialists promoting misinformation about HIV tests and antiretroviral drugs being the cause of AIDS.[53] Both Rath and Null sow disbelief and skepticism toward the medical establishment—what Dan Hurley describes as a "classic strategy used to promote belief in alternative remedies."[55] The Rath Health Foundation sells a range of vitamin remedies, whereas Gary Null pitches a wide set of holistic and nutritional products for AIDS.[55] AIDS activists, in turn, have sought to expose the cultropreneurs as charlatans, to educate people about why scientific testing is necessary, and, in the case of Rath, suing him successfully in South African courts.[56] In the case of Null, AIDS treatment activists have sought to keep his radio programs off mainstream channels precisely because of his promotion of AIDS denialists.[57]

It is telling that Duesberg has posted on his website an article by Null (written for *Penthouse*), which not only outlines Duesberg's critique of HIV science and antiretrovirals but also promotes a set of alternative therapies conveniently available from Null's sales outlets.[58] That Duesberg tolerates (and even promotes) cultropreneurs like Null speaks to the distance that has grown between him and the norms, values, and practices of the scientific community. And Duesberg appears to recognize this. As he told a reporter from *Newsweek*, "The whole dissident movement attracts a lot of crazies. . . . And then all of a sudden, without realising it, you have become one of them."[59]

One of the problems with becoming part of an oppositional culture (to mainstream science) is the difficulties involved in making clear distinctions between "crazy" and more plausible alternative therapies. As Campbell noted when describing the cultic milieu, the "common consciousness of deviance and the need to justify their own views in the light of the expressed ridicule or hostility of the larger society" gives rise to a "prevailing orientation of mutual sympathy and support such that the various cultic movements rarely engage in criticism of one another."[60] Perhaps Duesberg recognizes that AIDS denialism is effectively part of the cultic milieu and that tolerating cultropreneurs just goes with the territory. But if so, there is very little room for scientific methods or practices to engage with his ideas (see also chapter 7).

In line with the broader spiritualism common in the cultic milieu, a familiar refrain within AIDS denialism is that AIDS is caused by "stress" and harmful mental states. For example, Michael Ellner, the president of HEAL (Health Education AIDS Liaison)[61] who runs a "medical hypnosis" service,[62] argues that it is the HIV diagnosis itself that kills AIDS patients by pushing them into the "AIDS zone," his term for a collection of intense, chronic, and "very toxic emotional states," including shame and fear, which supposedly "knock out and undermine" the body's natural defenses.[63] Repairing their mental state is thus his solution to AIDS—a convenient prescription given his line of work.

Another member of HEAL is Roberto Giraldo, who not only sits on the boards of Rethinking AIDS and Alive and Well, but describes himself as a "natural health counsellor" and runs a clinic of "integral psycho immunology" in Brazil.[64] Infamous for advising Tshabalala-Msimang on nutritional alternatives to antiretrovirals (chapter 5), he subsequently went on to become the leading figure promoting organized AIDS denialism into Latin America. He has links with a Mexican AIDS denialist, Juan José Flores (also on the board of Alive and Well), who runs an organization called Vivo y Sano México, which makes similar claims about treating immune problems naturally.[66] The Mexican government became so alarmed by what they saw as the growing influence of AIDS denialists like Giraldo and Flores that several press conferences were held to warn people of the dangers of following their advice.[66]

Cultropreneurs, and indeed all alternative therapists, respond to challenges to the efficacy of their remedies by providing anecdotal evidence and testimonies of people who were satisfied with the treatment. In this respect, the role of the "living icon," the person who through his or her very existence "proves" that HIV disease can be fought with alternative remedies, is crucial. It is thus hardly surprising that Null produces videos featuring the "real" heroes of AIDS: those who have rejected antiretroviral treatment in favor of "cleansing," vitamin boosting, and taking herbal remedies.[67] The most important of these icons for the AIDS denialist movement was Christine Maggiore, the now deceased founder of Alive and Well, which supports "holistic" alternatives to antiretrovirals.

LIVING ICONS: PUTTING THEIR BODIES ON THE LINE

In the film, *The Other Side of AIDS*, Christine Maggiore says:

> In 1992 when I tested HIV-positive, I was told I had between five and seven years to live. Eight years later, I'm living in perfect health without any AIDS medicines. . . . The reason I have what I have today is because I did not follow doctor's orders. I questioned them. And I encourage all of you to question what you have been told about HIV and AIDS.[68]

Attractive, charismatic, and coherent, Maggiore was a central living icon for the AIDS denialist movement. In her writings, interviews, and public appearances, she disputed HIV science and campaigned against the use of antiretrovirals. She was strongly influenced by Duesberg and was one of several AIDS denialists invited to meet Mbeki in 2000.[69]

According to the preface of her widely distributed book, *What If Everything You Thought You Knew about AIDS Was Wrong*,[70] she lost faith in HIV science after a series of inconsistent HIV tests. This prompted her to conduct her own investigation "outside the confines of the AIDS establishment," which concluded that "AIDS research had jumped on a bandwagon that was headed in the wrong direction." Finding conventional AIDS groups unreceptive to the "life-affirming" information she found, Maggiore started her own organization, Alive and Well (including Duesberg on the board) to "share vital facts about HIV and AIDS that are unavailable from mainstream venues." Writing in 2000, she observed that her HIV status had been "decidedly positive" for five years, but that she was enjoying good health and was living "without pharmaceutical treatments or fear of AIDS."[71]

The saga of Maggiore's test results is a crucial foundational narrative for her as an AIDS denialist. The supposed inconsistencies in her test results are emblematic of her distrust in HIV science—and feature prominently in the AIDS denialist film *House of Numbers*. A standard AIDS denialist claim, explicated at length in this film, is that because different HIV tests (for the antigens, or for the antibodies, or for the viral load itself) can deliver different results, the entire edifice of AIDS science is flawed. Maggiore's test results are presented as a case in point

The first laboratory report shown in *House of Numbers* purporting to be Maggiore's first HIV test result is a positive Elisa test (for the presence of HIV antibodies) and a positive Western blot test (for HIV antigens) showing reactive bands for the p24 and gp120/160 antigens, but not for p31. The absence of p31 suggests either a relatively new HIV infection or a 4.8 percent chance of a false positive test—hence the correct procedure is to counsel patients that although they may be HIV infected, there is some doubt about the conclusion and thus further testing is necessary.[72] Indeed, this is what Maggiore appears to have been advised, and a further test was conducted. This, according to Maggiore, came back "indisputably positive," suggesting that her earlier test result probably indicated a recent HIV infection. Her doctor then reportedly told her that she had "five to seven" years to live, and that her only treatment options always resulted in the eventual use of AZT. Maggiore wrote, "I went directly from his office to a health food store" and the following day "began a search for a new AIDS specialist."[73]

She eventually found a doctor who, she says, "didn't routinely fill people with toxic pharmaceuticals and lethal predictions." This doctor persuaded her to do another test, which she says came back indeterminate, and then three more—which Maggiore reports came back positive, negative, and positive again. Evidence for the negative test result is unclear as the clip shown in *House of Numbers* focuses on a fragment of the test result showing nothing demonstrating a negative result. But when the film shows the final test result, it is clear that all bands on the Western blot are positive for HIV antigens—an unequivocally positive result. Maggiore concludes from her experience that HIV tests are "unreliable and inaccurate," yet the progression of her HIV tests from indeterminate to positive is consistent with her first test having been conducted soon after she became infected with HIV, with subsequent tests being performed in line with clinical practice and culminating in an unambiguously positive test result.[74]

Maggiore's book, endorsed by Duesberg, Rasnick, and Mullis, is a good illustration of AIDS denialist tactics. The first is to deny the evidence. Thus, in her section on antiretrovirals, she makes the baldly false statement that four years into the era of highly active antiretroviral treatment "there are still no reports in scientific journals that provide evidence for health improvement in patients taking these powerful drugs."[75] The second is to dismiss the evidence that does not suite the case: thus studies showing that CD4 counts improve for people on antiretroviral treatment are dismissed as dealing with "surrogate markers," and studies showing improved survival for patients on highly active antiretroviral treatment as opposed to AZT monotherapy are dismissed as not being placebo-controlled, i.e., as failing to have a control group that is given an inert substance rather than any medication.

Placebo-controlled trials, of course, are unethical if there is already a standard of care, which in the case of HIV disease was treatment with AZT. Which brings us to a third denialist trope (and one that proved compelling for Mbeki): extreme distrust of AZT. Maggiore points out, correctly, that AZT turned out to have transient benefits when used as a monotherapy, and that at the initially high doses prescribed, it had severe side effects.[76] But she rejects the scientific explanation for the eventual failure of AZT as a monotherapy (that the virus becomes resistant through mutation), simply by stating (again, obviously incorrectly) that there is no scientific evidence for the "mutation hypothesis."[77] Instead, she highlights the side effects of AZT, dismisses the other reverse transcriptase inhibitors as being "modelled after AZT," and disputes that there is any evidence for the benefits of protease inhibitors. In this respect, her argument draws heavily on Duesberg's and Rasnick's claims about antiretrovirals being "AIDS by prescription."

The fear and distrust of AZT are evidenced also in Maggiore's section on pregnancy and HIV, which raises concerns about toxicity and birth defects. Although the book does not recommend outright that HIV-positive women avoid MTCTP programs, the message any pregnant woman reading this section would get is that you should go nowhere near the conventional medical system because you may be falsely tested as HIV-positive and then forced to take a toxic drug that will cause birth defects in your baby. Instead, the message is rather to eat healthily and use alternative healing modalities (a long list of which is printed in her book, ranging from herbal therapies to homeopathy, "detoxifaction," and "imagery").

Maggiore, as Farber notes, "became a kind of motivational figurehead for the HIV positives of the world, speaking, holding meetings and working behind the scenes to help mothers and fathers who were under siege by draconian HIV mandates."[78] When she was pregnant in 2002 with her second child, Maggiore was featured on the cover of *Mothering* (a pro-alternative healing and anti-vaccination magazine) with a red circle slash symbol over the letters "AZT" emblazoned across her abdomen.[79] After her daughter, Eliza Jane Scovill, was born, Maggiore increased the risk of transmitting HIV yet further by breastfeeding the child. Tragically, Eliza Jane died in 2005 at age three of what the Los Angeles coroner ruled to be AIDS-related pneumonia.[80] Seven weeks earlier, Maggiore had stated on a radio show that her children have "excellent records of health,"[81] yet the coroner reported that Eliza Jane was underweight, under-height, and had pronounced atrophy of her thymus and other lymphatic organs. He found Pneumocystis jirovecii, a common AIDS-related opportunistic infection and leading cause of pediatric AIDS deaths[82] in her lungs and protein components of HIV (p24) in her brain.

Maggiore and her supporters, however, continued to deny that HIV had anything to do with the death, relying instead on a rival report by Alive and Well advisory board member Mohammed Al Bayati. Bayati is an animal toxicologist and was a co-applicant with Duesberg on his unsuccessful 1993 NIH AIDS-related grant application. He is neither a medical doctor nor board-certified in human pathology, yet consults on "health issues related to AIDS, adverse reactions to vaccines and medications" for $100 an hour.[83] According to him, Eliza Jane died because of an allergic reaction to an antibiotic (an absurd conclusion subsequently debunked by physician Nick Bennett).[84] Predictably, Maggiore and *Mothering* magazine agreed with Al Bayati.[85]

In Maggiore's eyes, it was Western medicine that killed Eliza Jane (rather than her own rejection of it): "the unfortunate irony in this situation is that the one time that we were asked to and we complied with mainstream medicine, we inadvertently gave our daughter something that took her life."[86] She also raised questions about the autopsy tests and dismissed the presence of p24 capsid protein in Eliza Jane's brain (a clear indication of HIV infection) as being the result of a "scavenger hunt" designed to make an HIV diagnosis.[87] In Farber's sympathetic account, the coroner went out of his way to make the death look like it was AIDS-related simply because she was Maggiore's child.[89] In similar conspiratorial vein, Farber attributed public anger—manifested in angry e-mails to Maggiore, web postings, and even printed flyers condemning her for Eliza Jane's death—to "the impossibly censorious and even brutal treatment one can expect if one is branded an 'AIDS denialist,'" concluding that AIDS has "become synonymous with rage and hatred of those who think differently from the orthodoxy." She wrote:

> I started to see the story as one that was less and less medical, more and more psycho-social—a story of an almost crushing kind of mob rule, where the victims have no rights. Few could resist the delicious temptation to condemn a "denialist" mother, or to appropriate EJ as their own tragic little girl. It was all done in the pitch-perfect tones of the AIDS morality play some of us know so well.[89]

Farber's argument is remarkable for its failure to consider that Eliza Jane was the victim in this instance, and that the "AIDS morality play" she sneers at is rooted in genuine social concern about the well-being of children. As Wainberg, the outspoken critic of AIDS denialism, puts it: "Maggiore was so misguided in believing this concoction of bullshit, that it cost not only her life, which is her business, but also the life of her three-year-old kid, and that is everybody's business."[90]

John Moore and I made a similar point, arguing in a *New York Times* editorial[91] that those who stand in positions of authority, be it the president of a country (Mbeki) or a parent, should not indulge their own intellectual questionings and reject the scientific consensus when it is others who pay the price. This prompted a subsequent e-mail exchange with Maggiore (later posted by Rethinking AIDS on the Internet)[92] which is illuminating for the way in which scientific evidence is immediately deflected by AIDS denialists with further questions—as if the questions themselves are sufficient to consign the evidence to irrelevance. Maggiore questioned our conclusion (based on the coroner's report) that Eliza Jane had died of AIDS and asked me to explain "how does Eliza Jane's eight-year-old brother, raised in the same manner as his sister, test HIV negative, along with my husband and partner of 10 years with whom I've had normal, latex-free relations?" She also disputed our observation that she was spreading "dangerous views" by claiming she was simply raising "unanswered questions" in the hope of being provided with "answers and references."

I subsequently provided her with references showing high death rates among untreated HIV-infected children and to the benefits of antiretroviral treatment in extending life[93] (and she predictably responded by stating that the drug trials were not placebo-controlled, that the HIV tests relied on "surrogate markers," and denying that there had been any scientific advance showing how HIV causes AIDS). When I argued that not all children born to HIV-positive mothers test negative, and hence that her son Charlie was one of the "lucky ones," she responded by asking for a "more cogent explanation than good fortune" for Charlie and her husband's HIV-negative status.

I also expressed the wish that

> When you reach the stage when HIV has undermined your immune system sufficiently to start causing you serious health problems, I sincerely hope that you start taking antiretroviral therapy. By all accounts, you are a good mother to Charlie, and it would be sad for him to lose you unnecessarily early. Three of the survey fieldworkers who work in my research centre

started antiretroviral treatment in the past two years and they are all doing very well—and one of them even gave birth to a (HIV-negative) child. This is all great cause for celebration and hope in this horrible epidemic.

She responded by pointing out that she was in her fourteenth year of living with HIV "with no medications and no health problems" and asking rhetorically, "How long do you suppose I might expect to continue in this way?" (Although Maggiore lived longer than average, she eventually progressed to AIDS and died three years later.)[94] With regard to my fieldworkers, she said:

> How do you measure "doing well"—clinical health, lab markers? I know a great number of HIV positive women who have given birth to HIV negative children without taking anti-HIV meds. The common factors among them are natural good health prior to testing positive, excellent nutrition, regular use of vitamin supplements, regular exercise, no use of AIDS meds, prescription drugs or street drugs, no smoking or drinking. Why are their experiences not "cause for celebration and hope" for a healthy, low cost alternative to toxic drugs whose long-term effects on mother or child remain unknown?

In other words, our exchange (in which the Rethinking AIDS leadership acted as advisers to Maggiore)[95] was clearly fruitless. It illustrates how people in denial can, as Kalichman observes, construct a reality that is "impenetrable by facts."[96] When Eliza Jane died, Maggiore told reporters: "I have been brought to my emotional knees, but not in regard to the science of this topic. . . . I am not second-guessing or questioning my understanding of the issue."[97] Maggiore remained in denial to the end, dying in 2009 at age 52 of bilateral bronchial pneumonia and disseminated herpes viral infection—both common AIDS-related opportunistic infections.[98] That she was prepared to endanger her own life, and that of her husband and children, speaks volumes about the passion and sincerity with which AIDS denialist beliefs can be embraced and to the powerful psychological forces at work.

AIDS activist Jeanne Bergman suggests that the phenomenon is understandable if we see AIDS denialism as a "kind of cult" replete with its own sense of persecution and spiritual enlightenment and even mystical powers.[99] She highlights the widespread AIDS denialist belief, evident also in Maggiore's own writings, that it is stress and fear itself that causes AIDS. Predictably, perhaps, Maggiore's supporters attributed her death to psychological stress (either resulting from the projections of worried friends or, as Farber put it, succumbing to the stress of the fight against the AIDS establishment: "I feared the battle would kill her, as I have felt it could kill me if I couldn't find enough beauty to offset the malevolence. This is a deeply occult battle, and Christine got caught in its darkest shadows."[100]

An autopsy was conducted on Maggiore by a professional independent pathologist, but the report was never released by the family. Instead, Al-Bayati offered an "interpretation" of it—namely that despite the presence of AIDS-defining conditions, Maggiore, like her daughter, had died of antibiotic poisoning.[101] Inevitably, conspiratorial moves were also made by Maggiore's supporters. For example, referring to himself as "Christine's private investigator," the retired police traffic officer and active AIDS denialist Clark Baker[102] claimed that "it is clear that corrupt officials from within the LA County Department of Health have pressured officials into making false claims that Maggiore and her daughter died of HIV so that pharmaceutical marketers could induce useful media idiots to perpetuate the myth on their behalf."[103]

The death of this important living icon was obviously a hard blow for organized AIDS denialism. One response is to brush this embarrassing fact under the carpet. Although Maggiore's organization Alive and Well posted a memorial notice when she died, visitors to the website today are still greeted with a "message" from Christine Maggiore on the "About Us" page, which gives no indication that she is dead.[104] Pro-science activists and anti–AIDS denialist sites (such as www.aidstruth.org, which lists the many AIDS denialists who have died)[105] by contrast reported her death as an illustration of the human costs of rejecting HIV science.[106] Other attempts have been made to create new "living icons"—for example, the people profiled on a website called "We are Living Proof."[107] The most active of these was Karri Stokely,[108] who made various public appearances and features in several YouTube videos. She died of pneumonia in April 2011 but continued to appear as if alive on the We are Living Proof website. But even when she was healthy, Stokely did not come close to what Maggiore offered in her capacity as living icon and central organizer for the movement.

Kalichman runs an anti-denialist website on which he posts news, criticisms of the AIDS denialists, and letters from members of the public. Here is an example of one of those letters, which speaks directly to Maggiore's symbolic status. The writer talks about how his "dissident" beliefs encouraged him to ignore his positive HIV test result, but that when he heard that Maggiore had died, alarm bells started ringing for him:

> In 2008 I had bumped into the website aidstruth.org and, while reading it in a "yeah blah blah whatever" kind of attitude, I saw the "denialists who have died" and "who the denialists are" sections. Something clicked. And very soon after I paid one of my usual visits to the Alive and Well site and found the memorial text about Maggiore's death. It didn't mention the cause (of course) so I Googled away thinking "please, let it be a traffic accident or something" and bam! Pneumonia . . .
>
> You know how denialists usually say it's just a coincidence, like "why not? Anybody can have pneumonia," but having recently read the list of dead denialists and wondering if those weren't too many untimely coincidences, for me Maggiore's death is where I drew the line. For me it was the "one too many" coincidence. That's where I secretly started to wonder if I had been wrong.[109]

Even so, he reports that it took a diagnosis of Kaposi's sarcoma before he rejected the AIDS denialist paradigm and started taking antiretrovirals, the pills he says he had been "indoctrinated to think of as pure evil."

In order to understand the dynamics of such "indoctrination," we need to pay some attention to the role of the praise-singers—the journalists and filmmakers who promote the cause of AIDS denialism by boosting the public profile of the hero scientists and living icons and publishing stories about the evils of antiretroviral treatment.

THE PRAISE-SINGERS

In his seminal account of the politics of AIDS science in the 1980s and early 1990s, Steven Epstein draws attention to how Duesberg was able to construct a rival social basis of authority by bypassing the scientific establishment and promoting his ideas directly to the public through the print and electronic media.[110] Duesberg was assisted in this task by a sizeable group of sympathetic journalists—their importance to him being reflected in the links he provides to their writings on his website.[111]

Chief among them is Celia Farber, who is thanked on the We Are Living Proof website as being the "person who has done more than anyone to share the truth with the world."[112] She started promoting the AIDS denialist cause in 1987 when she began writing and editing a monthly investigative feature column for *Spin* magazine called "Words from the Front" (1987–1995). It focused on the early critiques of HIV science and AZT.[113]

In 2006 she catapulted Duesberg back into the public eye in a piece for *Harper's* magazine[114]—prompting AIDS activists and researchers to set up www.aidstruth.org in order to post a rebuttal of her article.[115] Precisely because of the influence of praise-singers like Farber, AIDS activists have sought to contain it. For example, when it was learned that Duesberg and Farber were going to be presented with an award at 2008's "Washington Whistleblower Week,"[116] AIDS activist Richard Jefferys alerted the unsuspecting organizers about their stance on AIDS and the event was removed from the public program.[117] Anti–AIDS denial bloggers also challenge Farber online about her persistent misrepresentation of HIV science.[118]

Although she adopts the pose of an independent journalist, Farber is clearly hostile to HIV science, describing it in an interview as having been "co-opted by an almost industrial revolution of financial interest which clouded the truth and the data and the reality very powerfully and put new fears into the system."[119] In a 2010 web post, she argued that there was "no evidence" for a single germ causation model for AIDS and that

> All signs point to the importance of the intestinal tract, nutrition, fungal
> overload, and the importance of casting off the despair and fear imposed

by the Gallo/NCI theory and the Pharma-funded minions who continue to make tens of millions of dollars in reward for pushing drugs only and relentless persecution of those seeking other answers.

AIDS denialists, by contrast, are defended as "ethical, brave human beings" while AIDS activists are castigated for deploying "abuse, debasement, slander, lies, professional assassination, espionage and McCarthyism all in the name of wanting to 'save lives.'"[120]

Journalism and blogging are important sources of publicity for AIDS denialism, but video is becoming an increasingly powerful medium, as witnessed by the many clips on YouTube posted by cultropreneurs like Gary Null and "documentaries" made by independent filmmakers which are shown in film festivals and even on television. These include *The Other Side of AIDS*, *Guinea Pig Kids* by Jamie Doran, and *House of Numbers* by Brent Leung.

Of these, *Guinea Pig Kids* (2004) garnered the most publicity because the story it told spoke to long-standing concerns within the African-American community about medical trials and abuse of power by the authorities. The story deals with the inclusion of HIV-positive foster children from New York City in antiretroviral drug trials during the late 1980s and 1990s, i.e., at a time when access to drug trials was often the only way to obtain treatment. Largely as a result of pressure from pediatricians, children (including foster children) were enrolled in trials of antiretrovirals which had already been tested in adults, but for which pediatric formulations were being developed. The Incarnation Children's Center, a small, specialized care facility for HIV-infected foster children, was included in the trials. The trials were initially for AZT, but shifted to the multiple-drug cocktails and protease inhibitors from the 1990s as the standard of care changed. "To deny these kids the medications would have been a crime," said Dr. William Caspe, chairman of pediatrics at Jacobi Medical Center in the Bronx. "Because of what we did, we were able to keep them alive until newer medications became available."[121] The AIDS denialists, however, thought otherwise.

Apparently "tipped off" and assisted by Maggiore,[122] Liam Scheff investigated the story and wrote "The House That AIDS Built," which he placed online at indymedia.org—a website describing itself as an "outlet for radical, accurate and passionate telling of the truth"—after failing to publish it elsewhere.[123] The story complained about drug toxicity, the force-feeding of medications to children, side effects, and deaths. This came to the attention of Vera Sharav, founder of the Alliance for Human Research Protection, who is opposed to the participation of children in clinical trials.[124] She laid a charge with the FDA and the federal Office for Human Research Protections. At the same time, the *New York Post* ran a series of articles with headlines such as "AIDS Tots Used as Guinea Pigs." Independent filmmaker Doran enlisted Scheff, Sharav, and Farber to help him make *Guinea Pig Kids*, which was aired on BBC2 in November 2004. That the film was seriously biased is evident by its reliance on David Rasnick for its "expert" commentary on antiretroviral treatment.

The reports alarmed African-American activists and politicians in the city, particularly Omowale Clay, a leader of the December 12th Movement, a Brooklyn-based group that campaigns for reparations for slavery and acts as a watchdog group for civil rights violations. He told journalists that "98% of the children experimented on were black and Latino and that the fundamental basis of why they chose those kids was racism. They have the arrogance to say it was for their own good, but we know it was racism."[125] Clay showed *Guinea Pig Kids* in churches, block association meetings, and private gatherings—and, along with several city councilmen, called for council hearings and an investigation by the city.

The issue was ripe for suspicion because the medical trial records were incomplete, in part because many different agencies and organizations were involved at different times and the city's Administration for Children's Services (ACS) had been through four changes in administration since the trials began. Fuel was added to the fire when the ACS discovered additional documentation in its basement indicating that 465 children, rather than the 89 it originally claimed, had participated in HIV-related clinical trials, although most were not at the Incarnation Children's Center. The ACS commissioned the Vera Institute of Justice to review the evidence (at a cost of $1.5 million), and other investigations were conducted into whether the guidelines for including foster children in trials had been violated. When the child welfare commissioner John Mattingly testified about the trials at a city council hearing, angry spectators shouted him down, invoking the specter of Tuskegee. As journalists Jannie Scott and Leslie Kaufman observe, the outcome demonstrated

> the power of a single person armed only with access to the Internet and an incendiary story to put major institutions on the defensive. The story taps a combustible mix of fears: the suspicions of some activists that AIDS is not necessarily caused by HIV and that AIDS drugs do not necessarily help, and the belief of some black people that the medical establishment does not always have their interests at heart.[126]

According to one report, the heated rhetoric subsided "as the agenda of Maggiore and Scheff became better known"[127] and after the BBC retracted the documentary in May 2007 following an investigation. This investigation was sparked by complaints by AIDS activists and HIV scientists, notably Jeanne Bergman and John Moore, about the biased and inaccurate reporting. Ironically, Rethinking AIDS played into the hands of the complainants when David Crowe released a press statement praising the documentary— thereby allowing John Moore to bring the clear link between AIDS denialism and the documentary to the attention of the BBC.[128]

The BBC investigation found that Doran's documentary had breached its standards of accuracy (and posted a correction, distancing the broadcaster from the film).[129] In 2009 the Vera Institute of Justice released its report.[130] It found that there was no evidence that any child died because of the trials or had been selected for the trials on the basis of race. For Liam Scheff, this was simply further evidence of a broad conspiracy to silence criticism of the AIDS industry.[131]

The documentary film House of Numbers (2009) made the rounds of minor film festivals (even picking up a few awards) but was panned by reviews in the mainstream press. Unlike Guinea Pig Kids, which gained traction by resonating with medical mistrust in the black community, House of Numbers focused on HIV science, projecting it as fundamentally divided, unreliable, and corrupt. The film shows Mullis accusing the US Centers for Disease Control and Prevention as having been looking for a new plague in order "scare" the American people into giving them more money, and Duesberg likening HIV scientists to "prostitutes." It also raises the usual AIDS denialist questions about HIV tests and so on, prompting Jeanne Bergman to collate and post a set of "real answers" to his "fake questions."[132] Ben Goldacre (a doctor and pro-science writer) was also incensed enough to comment about the film's duplicity—especially the way it starred Maggiore without reporting her daughter's death, and only mentioning "in the last 2 seconds of the film, at the end of the lengthy credits, in small letters" that she herself had died.[133]

Leung was able to interview many leading HIV scientists, projecting himself as a naive and neutral questioner on a voyage of discovery. He is, however, anything but. Not only was he involved in a prior video project with Boyd Graves (chapter 2), but *House of Numbers* was funded at least in part by Rethinking AIDS. The minutes from a meeting in 2006 reveal that motions proposed by Leppo and Giraldo (and seconded by Maggiore) were passed unanimously that funding be allocated to Leung for the film.[134] Neither this nor other sources of funding are acknowledged in the film or on its website.

HIV SCIENTISTS FIGHT BACK

The HIV scientists who were interviewed in the film were angry with the way Leung cut and presented their interviews. Several of them released statements condemning the film.[135] John Moore posted the following comment in a debate on the web pages of the *Spectator*.[136]

> I'm one of the scientists (the legitimate ones) that Leung deceived into appearing in this shoddy film. He used Sasha Baron Cohen-style tactics to sit in our offices and disguise his true agenda—as "honest investigation"? Yeah, right. . . . Leung is an AIDS denialist, pure and unadulterated. And his multi-million dollar [film] and its promotional budget was paid for by a few wealthy AIDS denialist backers that Leung consistently refuses to identify (so much for full and frank disclosure of funding sources, expected of and honored by AIDS scientists, but ignored by those who criticize them).

> The film itself is deliberately edited to make AIDS scientists look bad, and to create controversy where none lies. And of course Leung's friends are made to look wise and thoughtful, honest questioners of the truth, when the reality is very, very different. . . .
>
> There is much material on the AIDS denialists, who they are and what they do, posted on the AIDS Truth website. Read it and weep that such crazy and evil people can still influence others to make poor choices with their lives.

This resulted in a slew of counter-posts in which John Moore was accused of being in the pay of the pharmaceutical industry. These were subsequently determined to be libelous and removed by the *Spectator* (which also agreed to compensate Moore by making a donation to an AIDS charity—Moore nominated the Treatment Action Campaign).

One of those the slick film initially impressed was Caspar Melville, editor of the *New Humanist,* who described it as raising important questions and leaving him "armed with a greater understanding of issues pertinent to AIDS and HIV."[137] However, after talking to Leung and finding out more about AIDS denialism (something he was prompted to do after being chastised by Ben Goldacre),[138] Melville concluded that *House of Numbers* was actually an "insidious interweaving of interviews with 'the establishment' that makes their position look arrogant or incoherent (or is edited to make them agree with the film's thesis) and interviews with 'expert witnesses' who turn out to all be representatives of one view (if not organisation) and whose expertise is questionable if not non-existent."[139]

Melville's posting sparked a long set of comments, some from AIDS denialists questioning his about-fact, but most from activist doctors (such as Nick Bennett, a member of www.aidstruth.org who runs his own anti–AIDS denialist website)[140] and individuals like J. T. de Shong[141] and "Snout,"[142] who run similar anti-denial blogs and engage frequently in online combat with AIDS denialists. Gus Cairns, editor of a major HIV newsletter, *HIV Treatment Update,* contributed to the comment string by pointing out that antiretrovirals had saved his life:

> In the early 1990s, having been diagnosed in 1985, I refused to take AZT and put myself on a programme of vitamin supplements, Chinese medi-

cine, psychotherapy, yoga, swimming with dolphins—you name it. None of it made the slightest difference. By late 1996 I had a CD4 count of 10 (i.e., 1% of the normal complement), numerous AIDS-related illnesses, and had lost 25% of my body weight. The only thing that made a difference was to take a supposedly toxic cocktail of antiretrovirals, which I started in January 1997. My CD4 count immediately improved, my illnesses faded away, and here I am.

Predictably, others countered his post by claiming that they were living proof that antiretrovirals were toxic and that one could live well without them. This prompted Kalichman to observe that this showed how AIDS denialists live in a different universe, one that psychiatrists call "an encapsulated delusion."[143] Kalichman also wrote to Melville telling him not to feel bad about being conned because the AIDS denialists are a "mix of narcissists and conmen" and it is "extremely easy to buy into their crap."[144]

In his book, *Denying AIDS*, Kalichman writes about how angry he became when a colleague told him that she was not prepared to act as a reviewer for *AIDS and Behavior* (the academic journal he edits) because she agreed with Duesberg. He attributes his anger and subsequent decision to become more active on the issue to the harm that AIDS denialism can cause:

> Reading that HIV does not cause AIDS can dissuade people from getting tested for HIV, lead HIV infected people to ignore their HIV positive test result, and persuade some to reject antiretroviral therapies in place of vitamins and nutritional supplements. These are not hypothetical situations. Real people are facing a life threatening disease that can be effectively treated. Realizing that all AIDS scientists should take action to counter the claims of HIV/AIDS denialism, I decided to write this book.[145]

As part of this activism, Kalichman joined other HIV scientists in taking action against a journal for publishing a paper by Duesberg without first subjecting it to peer review. Chapter 7 takes up this story.

7

DEFENDING THE IMPRIMATUR
OF SCIENCE

This chapter considers the way the scientific community has responded to Peter Duesberg's AIDS denialism. Particular attention is paid to the action taken against the journal *Medical Hypotheses* for publishing a paper by Duesberg and others without first subjecting it to meaningful editorial review. The episode highlights the importance of peer review as a core scientific value. But because Duesberg's paper defended Mbeki's stance on AIDS (by claiming there is no real AIDS epidemic in Africa and that antiretrovirals are harmful), the consequences for public health of publishing poor scholarship in a seemingly "scientific" journal were very much at the foreground in this dispute.

The term *scientific community* is suggestive of old Mertonian ideas of organized skepticism, i.e., an enquiring, empirically oriented intellectual society committed to, and governed by, norms of reason and universalism.[1] Sociologists of science have since shown that the social character of science is more profound than implied in American sociologist Robert K. Merton's original conception—that who gets to practice and produce science is shaped by networks of power and prestige[2] and that different "evidential cultures" exist with regard to the interpretation of data and management of disputes over it.[3] Even so, broad communal norms, such as respect for evidence and peer review, remain very much in evidence and can spark genuine moral outrage when violated. This was the case with regard to the *Medical Hypotheses* saga when HIV scientists and activists engaged in "boundary work" in defense of peer review as a core scientific value.

BOUNDARY WORK AND EDITORIAL REVIEW

According to Thomas Gieryn, "boundary work" refers to the "practical, ideological activity" undertaken by scientists to defend and demarcate what counts as scientific, the crucial point being that such activities have "real implications for status, authority, career opportunities and resources."[4] He argued that the boundaries of what is understood as "science" do not depend on obvious methodological distinctions, but are "drawn and redrawn in flexible, historically changing and sometimes ambiguous ways," depending on what particular interests are being pursued.[5] The *Medical Hypotheses* saga is an example of boundary work in that scientists took action against the publisher because the journal was not peer-reviewed, and hence, they argued, it should not count as scientific and should no longer be listed under Medline or have the scientific status of being searchable through PubMed. However, in contrast to Gieryn's interest-driven interpretation of why boundary work is undertaken, this episode suggests that it was moral outrage about the social costs of Duesberg's intransigence which prompted the action.

The contestation between Duesberg and HIV science is not simply one of rival truth claims. That Duesberg ignores counter-evidence and has no relevant expertise in HIV is important for understanding why the struggle took the form of attacking a journal for publishing one of his papers, rather than engaging with the paper itself. The so-called "debate" between Duesberg and HIV scientists is not a debate at all, but rather, as Martin Weinel puts it, a "counterfeit scientific controversy."[6] That Duesberg is not engaging in a scientific manner on HIV is at the root of the problem.

Two normative issues are evident in the *Medical Hypotheses* saga: anger at Duesberg for ignoring HIV science and contributing to, and subsequently defending, Mbeki's AIDS policy tragedy; and anger at the way in which *Medical Hypotheses*, which has the façade of a scientific journal, was seen as inappropriately giving Duesberg's article the status of being scientific, even though it was published without adequate editorial review.

Editorial review has long been regarded as a core scientific practice which assists the process of quality control (albeit imperfectly), accreditation, and reputation-building.[7] As John Ziman put it evocatively, an article in a reputable scientific journal "does not merely represent the opinions of its author; it bears the imprimatur of scientific authenticity."[8] Different models of editorial review evolved over the past three centuries of scientific publishing. But since the expansion of academic research and growing specialization in the postwar period, peer review (i.e., review by referees other than the editor) has become standard.[9] While there was, and remains, concern that peer review may at times be inimical to the publication of revolutionary ideas,[10] that reviewers can be "mean spirited, lead-footed, capricious toadies and hacks,"[11] and that the "status hierarchy of science" influences the way authors write and how referees assess articles,[12] its consolidation as a core academic practice reflects a general judgment that its usefulness to the scientific community outweighs its costs. Different forms of peer review are continuing to evolve in an effort to overcome some of the limitations of traditional peer review. These range from open peer review requiring reviews to be signed, to posting submitted papers on preprint servers to elicit online comments and reviews, enabling authors to carry reviews from one journal to another, posting reviewer comments alongside the published paper, and running traditional peer-review processes simultaneously with a public review.[13] But even avant-garde facilities such as arXiv, an online open-access resource which posts papers (mainly in physics and the quantitative sciences) if they are topical and follow accepted standards of scholarly communication, have not overcome the need for peer review as a form of accreditation: 90 percent of the papers posted there are also submitted to traditional journals for publication.[14]

Medical Hypotheses, however, deliberately bucked the system. It was founded in 1975 by David Horobin explicitly as a non-peer-reviewed journal on the grounds that peer review necessarily suppressed "radical ideas" and was "wide open to serious abuse"[15] Its editorial policy mandated the editor to select articles on the basis of "potential importance and interest," using "broad criteria of scientific plausibility" where even "probably untrue papers" could be published if deemed to be "stimulating to the development of future science." In his founding editorial, Horobin argued that there was a need for this kind of journal in biomedical science because "ignorant and pedantic referees and editors" objected too quickly to what they saw as "unjustified speculation."[16] Taking up the mantle of what he believed to be progressive science, Horobin dedicated his journal to publishing ideas and speculations from "anyone regardless of whether they have done experimental work in the field or not." He declared:

> I shall publish some ideas which seem improbable and perhaps even faintly ridiculous. . . . Many, and probably most of the hypotheses published in this journal will turn out in some way to be wrong. But if they stimulate determined experimental testing, progress is inevitable whether they are wrong or right. Moreover the history of science has repeatedly shown that when hypotheses are proposed it is impossible to predict which will turn out to be revolutionary and which ridiculous. The only safe approach is to let all see the light and to let all be discussed, experimented upon, vindicated or destroyed.[17]

The problem with this position, of course, is that even if peer review represses revolutionary ideas, it does not follow that publishing "improbable" and "faintly ridiculous" ideas without peer review is the solution. In the absence of peer review, how are we to judge the credibility of work in any area beyond our own narrow areas of expertise? And if a journal becomes known for publishing ridiculous ideas, why would scientists subsequently bother to test and engage with them?

The issue of credibility through peer review came up in an e-mail exchange[18] between Duesberg, David Crowe (head of Rethinking AIDS), and Randall Scalise, a physicist who teaches a course at Southern Methodist University (Dallas) called "Debunking Pseudoscience."[19] Crowe had written to Scalise (copied to Duesberg) suggesting that he invite "dissidents" to discuss why "HIV is very unlikely to be the cause of AIDS." Scalise replied by asking: "Got anyone who has published this remarkable theory in the peer-reviewed medical literature in the last five years?" Duesberg then responded by asking Scalise to be more tolerant of scientific minorities because "all scientific innovation came from minorities, e.g., Galileo, Planck, Einstein." Scalise then pointed out that "Galileo's nemesis was the Roman Catholic Church, not other scientists" and that "Galileo, Planck, and Einstein are famous and respected because they published and in this way convinced their peers that they were correct."

Precisely because scientists are usually experts in narrow fields of study, they necessarily rely on peer opinion in other areas—and are especially alert to whether claims have been published in reputable, peer-reviewed journals or not. For all its faults, peer review remains an essential mechanism for the allocation of trust in the results of others. Indeed, precisely because it was not peer-reviewed, *Medical Hypotheses* failed to attain any authority or respect in the scientific community. And once Bruce Charlton assumed the editorship of *Medical Hypotheses*, the content became so eccentric that the journal became an object of ridicule.[20]

Medical Hypotheses was effectively ignored by mainstream scientists until, with the publication of Duesberg's article defending Mbeki's stance on AIDS, it was deemed by some to have become a danger to public health and action was taken to change the editorial policy of the journal or have it dropped from the stable of scientific journals. The story is told in more detail below, paying particular attention to the normative issues and responses of journal editors.

PETER DUESBERG, AIDS DENIALISM, AND THE SCIENTIFIC COMMUNITY

In late 2008 an article was published in the *Journal of Acquired Immune Deficiency Syndromes* (*JAIDS*) by Pride Chigwedere and colleagues arguing that 330,000 South Africans had died between 2000 and 2005 because President Mbeki delayed the provision of antiretrovirals in the public sector.[21] This estimate reinforced earlier South African work suggesting that 343,000 people had died of AIDS unnecessarily during the Mbeki presidency.[22] Both papers implicated AIDS denialists like Duesberg, who had served on Mbeki's Presidential AIDS Advisory Panel, and calls were made by activists to hold Mbeki and Duesberg to account.[23]

In his reply Duesberg and his coauthors defended Mbeki's stance in two ways, both of which denied or ignored the relevant science.[24] They argued that AIDS deaths in Africa were far lower than typically estimated (because they looked only at AIDS deaths actually registered on death certificates as such, while ignoring the many more deaths classified by AIDS-related opportunistic infections) and repeated Duesberg's decades-old claims that HIV does not cause AIDS and that "toxic" antiretroviral drugs are unnecessary and harmful. Chigwedere subsequently coauthored a detailed critique of this paper,[25] which was predictably dismissed by AIDS denialists as "part of an empire that is destroying lives through the pronouncement of death sentences, the use of toxic drugs and the demonization of gay men, Africans and the association of sex with terror, shame and death."[26]

Duesberg's claims have been systematically countered many times over the past twenty-five years,[27] yet he ignores these papers and continues to promote his assertions, unchanged and with increasingly outdated academic references.[28] This has made him a pariah in the scientific community not simply because he violates the norms of evidence-based science, but because his stance is unreasonable and ultimately insulting to other scientists. Maintaining hypotheses by ignoring strong evidence to the contrary not only undermines the possibility of scientific progress, but threatens the social basis of science itself. Respect for the evidence and for the people who generate it is essential for the functioning of the scientific community— and it is precisely this that Duesberg flouts. Warren Winkelstein, one of the early HIV epidemiologists, recalls how, at a meeting of the National Academy of Sciences in Washington to discuss Duesberg's theories, Duesberg would frequently get up, wander around the room, and start talking to reporters. In his view, Duesberg simply "wasn't listening to what was being said."[29] Scientists interpreted his message then, and continue to do so today, that Duesberg's "premises are based not on facts but on faith: faith that he is right, and that everyone else is wrong."[30]

Duesberg's reputation in the scientific community has been so damaged by his intransigence on AIDS that when *Scientific American* published an article by him on cancer,[31] the editors posted the following disclaimer alongside the article:

> The author, Peter Duesberg, a pioneering virologist, may be well known to readers for his assertion that HIV is not the cause of AIDS. The biomedical community has roundly rebutted that claim many times. Duesberg's ideas about chromosomal abnormality as a root cause for cancer, in contrast, are controversial, but are being actively investigated by mainstream science. We have therefore asked Duesberg to explain that work here. This article is in no sense an endorsement by *Scientific American* of his AIDS theories.

The disclaimer is noteworthy for the distinction it draws between controversial views in a legitimate debate (defined as one that is being "actively investigated by mainstream science") and intransigent views flying in the face of rebuttals. Duesberg and his supporters, of course, regard *any* closure on the "debate" about HIV not being the cause of AIDS as oppressive and ultimately "unscientific." The disclaimer in *Scientific American*, however, reflects the broader view within the HIV scientific community that Duesberg is no longer engaging on AIDS as a scientist.

A similar stance was adopted by John Maddox, the editor of *Nature*, thirteen years earlier when he concluded that Duesberg no longer had the "right of reply" in his journal. At that time, early studies of the HIV status of stored samples of donor blood and the development of AIDS among those who had received blood transfusions showed clear correlations between HIV infection and AIDS.[32] Duesberg, however, refused to accept this evidence for the connection between HIV-infected blood transfusions and subsequent AIDS deaths among hemophiliacs—and posited a set of alternative unfounded speculations (about potentially contaminated clotting factors) as the cause of such deaths.[33] Maddox became infuriated with Duesberg and, in an unprecedented editorial in *Nature*, announced that he would no longer be publishing Duesberg's letters and papers on the topic because of his unacceptable debating techniques, misreading of the work of others, and refusal to accept evidence contrary to his hypotheses.[34]

Maddox also complained about the way Duesberg "advertises" his position to the public, "thus giving many infected people the belief that HIV infection is not in itself the calamity it is likely to prove."[35] In a bolded line right under the title of his editorial, Maddox wrote: "Dr. Peter Duesberg, the virologist-turned-campaigner, is wrongly using tendentious arguments to confuse understanding of AIDS and those in danger of contracting the disease. He should stop." As such, Maddox's editorial was a prequel of the public health concerns that motivated the action against *Medical Hypotheses* sixteen years later.

BOUNDARY WORK AGAINST *MEDICAL HYPOTHESES*

When *JAIDS* published estimates by Chigwedere and others[36] of the human costs of Mbeki's AIDS policies, Duesberg submitted a coauthored reply to *JAIDS*, but it was rejected after peer review.[37] The paper was then submitted to *Medical Hypotheses*, where it was accepted within two days.

One of the *JAIDS* reviewers had complained about the paper's selective "cherry picking" and misrepresentation of scientific facts.[38] The reviewer drew particular attention to the misrepresentation of a *Lancet* paper[39] which showed that antiretroviral treatment reduced mortality significantly amongst AIDS patients, but that no *additional* improvement in mortality reduction had occurred between the late 1990s and early 2000s. Duesberg and his coauthors misrepresented this study by claiming that it showed that antiretrovirals do not decrease mortality *at all* and hence have no benefit.[40] This was, indeed, a blatant misrepresentation. Yet despite being alerted to the problem (which the reviewer suggested was serious enough to amount to scientific misconduct), Duesberg and his coauthors chose not to correct the text before sending it to *Medical Hypotheses*.

In defending his decision to publish Duesberg's paper, Bruce Charlton said he did so because it was in line with the journal's editorial policy and because "Duesberg is obviously a competent scientist, he is obviously the victim of an orchestrated campaign of intimidation and exclusion and I interpret his sacrifice of status to principle as *prima facie* evidence of his sincerity."[41] He argued that those who disagreed with Duesberg and others in his camp should have written letters and papers "countering the ideas and evidence presented" because this is "how real science is supposed to work."[42] The obvious problem with his analysis, though, is that Duesberg's arguments *had* been countered many times before (including by the *JAIDS* reviewers), with no apparent effect. The problem is not the absence of debate, but Duesberg's inability to acknowledge or respond to his critics. At the very least he should have corrected the obvious misrepresentation of the *Lancet* study. Charlton also sidesteps the impact of AIDS denialism on public health, i.e., the very issue that motivated the boundary work against his journal.

That Mbeki was able to justify delaying the use of antiretrovirals because a "scientific debate" was supposedly in need of resolution raised the thorny issue of whether scientists should have dignified or legitimated this stance by agreeing to serve on his Presidential AIDS Advisory Panel alongside AIDS denialists like Duesberg. After the two independent estimates had been published of how many people had died unnecessarily of AIDS during Mbeki's presidency because of his opposition to antiretrovirals,[43] *Nature* published an editorial criticizing the mainstream scientists for agreeing to serve on Mbeki's panel in the first place. The editorial argued that as there was "no possibility of consensus being reached among the panel's two diametrically opposed camps," that "in retrospect, the panel constituted as it was, should never have been supported."[44] Several scientists subsequently admitted that they had underestimated the strength of Mbeki's AIDS denialism, but defended their participation on the grounds that they believed they were doing their duty and had hoped "rationality would prevail."[45]

In any event, by the time Duesberg published his reply in *Medical Hypotheses*, the ideas that AIDS denialists were a threat to public health—and that it was pointless debating them—had wide currency in the scientific community. This helps us understand why the response to Duesberg took not only the form of a subsequent rebuttal[46] but also boundary work against *Medical Hypotheses* for publishing his flawed paper. More specifically, scientists and AIDS treatment activists wrote to the National Library of Medicine (NLM) requesting that *Medical Hypotheses* be reviewed for deselection from Medline on the grounds that articles were not adequately reviewed and that it had a disturbing track record of publishing pseudoscience and poor scholarship, especially on AIDS.[47]

The complainants argued that *Medical Hypotheses* did not meet the standards set for Medline-indexed journals because there was "no evidence of editorial oversight in the traditional sense of suggesting changes and revisions to ensure or improve quality" and that the journal's median time between submission and acceptance of three days "cannot be conducive to maintenance of journal quality, particularly in the absence of a peer review process." They also noted that articles were essentially editorials and that the journal had developed a reputation for "trivial and occasionally offensive content with no obvious relation to genuine medical research" (for example, papers on masturbation as a cure for congestion, high heels as a cause of schizophrenia, and on alleged similarities between Asian populations and people with Down syndrome). Their key criticism, however, was that *Medical Hypotheses* had become a "tool for the legitimization of at least one pseudoscientific movement with aims antithetical to the public health goals of the NIH and the NLM," notably AIDS denialism: "*Medical Hypotheses*, with its lack of peer review and careful editorial oversight, has published numerous articles advancing AIDS denialism allowing individual denialists, none of whom has ever published original research on HIV, to claim legitimacy as HIV researchers because their work has, after all, appeared in a 'scientific' journal." They go on to argue in connection to the Duesberg paper in particular that "the false claims in this paper were not vetted by the editor of *Medical Hypotheses* and that the journal, by publishing this and similar papers, has contributed significantly to the spread of medical misinformation and loss of life and wellbeing."

The NLM responded by promising to consider the matter, but in the meantime another group of scientists, including John Moore and Françoise Barré-Sinoussi, wrote to Elsevier, the publisher of *Medical Hypotheses*, about the letter to the NLM and to register further complaints about Duesberg's paper. They also wrote to their university libraries requesting that subscriptions to *Medical Hypotheses* be canceled and encouraged others to do so too—thereby prompting a broader "Cancel your *Medical Hypotheses* subscription" campaign with its own Facebook page.

How should we understand this episode of boundary work? Was it primarily in defense of power and privilege as suggested in Gieryn's original conceptualization of the term? This seems implausible. HIV science is sufficiently strong, both in terms of scientific productivity and access to resources, that the views of fringe AIDS denialists pose no threats to anyone's reputation or resources. Similarly, articles published in *Medical Hypotheses* carried no risk to their authors' reputations precisely because the journal lacked credibility in the scientific community. There were, in short, no immediate professional interests to be protected or advanced by the boundary work against *Medical Hypotheses*. Rather, their action was rooted in normative concerns—notably, potential harm to the public.

This is evident in a posting on September 12, 2009, by John Moore as part of a debate on Ben Goldacre's Bad Science blog about *Medical Hypotheses*:

> It harms nobody if *Medical Hypotheses* publishes papers on the Loch Ness Monster or the length of lines on palms. . . . But when it comes to AIDS denialism and the vaccine-autism allegations, lines are crossed because people ARE harmed. As scientists, we CANNOT live in Ivory Towers and natter away about our "rights" to publish anything and everything we want, whatever the consequences. Those rights are actually privileges, ones that are, in effect, granted to us by the public who fund what we do. We should respect that and act accordingly.[48]

Elsevier acted quickly after receiving the complaints. An expert panel was commissioned which recommended that the Duesberg paper be subject to external peer review. A subsequent peer-review process managed by the *Lancet's* editorial team unanimously recommended rejection, and Elsevier permanently withdrew the paper.[49] Charlton was instructed to introduce peer review or face termination of his contract as editor. He chose the latter course, depicting Elsevier's move as anti-science: "We have seen the destruction of the last non-peer-reviewed journal—the only one outside the normal power structures of science. . . . This is something new to science, indeed it is not science at all—as science was done in its golden age."[50]

Charlton also provided several spirited defenses of his stance in newspapers[51] and on blog postings. When Goldacre argued on Bad Science that *Medical Hypotheses* should not have published Duesberg's paper because it was "plainly foolish,"[52] Charlton posted a response saying he was "agnostic about the truth or correctness of the papers chosen for publication." Gold-acre replied by asking what possible justification there was for publishing an article that misrepresented a key reference (i.e., the study published in the *Lancet*):[53]

> This isn't a matter of perspective, or free expression of ideas, and it's not a disagreement of interpretation: it's a simple error of fact, they just misrepresented a key reference. What is your justification for publishing that and how does it fit into any kind of meaningful vision that can help ideas be disseminated and improved?

Charlton responded simply by restating the editorial policy of *Medical Hypotheses* and noting that "scientists and thinkers of real achievement" supported the journal. Seth Kalichman then took issue with him, arguing in his capacity as editor of *AIDS and Behavior* that peer review was important because science is stronger when undertaken as a collective exercise:

> one person, no matter how broadly trained, cannot make the call on every paper. . . . If your decisions were guided by expert opinions you would be less inclined to make such horrific errors in judgment. To be sure, peer review is not perfect, but it is far better than the beliefs of any one of us.[54]

One could interpret Kalichman's and Moore's arguments with Charlton as self-justificatory in that both could be seen as defending their being signatories to the letter to Elsevier, or their editorial work for peer-reviewed journals, or even their substantial contributions to the HIV/AIDS literature. But this would be too narrowly instrumental and disregards the important moral framing both lend to their comments. Both Kalichman and Moore believe that the methods employed by the scientific community to accredit knowledge, while far from flawless, are nevertheless the best we have for assessing rival truth claims. They are clearly outraged by the notion that a journal editor could be unconcerned about the truth status of the papers he publishes. For them, this is both an intellectual and a moral failure.

The exchange with Charlton over peer review is also interesting for the lack of dialogue between the opposing "sides." Charlton never tackles the substantive point—how to justify the publication of a paper, aspects of which are manifestly false. Instead he retreats to what is ultimately a relativist and subjective stance: the truth status of a paper is irrelevant, it is whether it is potentially interesting (in his eyes) that matters. And, by talking in conspiratorial terms about ideas and papers being "suppressed," he shifts the argument into a zone in which debate becomes impossible: precisely because papers are not being published elsewhere, this is seen as evidence of oppression and a valid reason for their publication in *Medical Hypotheses*. Whether a paper contains clear misrepresentations and factual errors is of no relevance when the situation is constructed in these terms.

CONCLUSION

The boundary work against *Medical Hypotheses* successfully asserted the importance of peer review in defining what counts as "scientific." Faced with the choice of changing the editorial policy of *Medical Hypotheses* or facing its possible removal from Medline listings, Elsevier opted to keep the journal within the scientific stable and require a stronger process of review.[55] The normative context, notably the demonstrable connection between AIDS denialism and hundreds of thousands of deaths in South Africa, probably made the decision easier.

But in the process some concerns were raised about the "silencing" of critical voices and its implications for both scientific research and academic freedom. *Science* published letters on both sides of the argument, and even the popular press got involved. For example, an editorial in the (London) *Times Higher Education* argued that academic freedom to hold unconventional views "can never be prized above life itself" but concluded that the way forward is "not to silence people such as Professor Duesberg or to change *Medical Hypotheses*, but for science to police its territory effectively and scientists to challenge papers on their science and debunk them forcefully, point by dangerous point."[56] How science can "police its territory effectively" without peer review is not confronted directly—and neither is the challenge of debating a position that has been debunked many times, without any apparent impact. And while noting that academic freedom should never be prized above life itself, the editorial refrains from commenting on how the scientific community ought to manage possible conflict between these objectives.

But does the withdrawal of Duesberg's paper and the introduction of peer review at *Medical Hypotheses* really imply that Duesberg and other "unconventional thinkers" have been "silenced"? No. To confuse peer review with an assault on academic freedom is to commit a category mistake. Duesberg is still free to promote his views and publish them wherever he can, including on the Internet. Maddox's action back in 1993 was much more of a problem for Duesberg because the Internet did not exist, and letters and articles in journals were necessary in terms of getting one's views "out there." But in today's electronic world, nobody can be "silenced" in any meaningful way (short of government's imposing blunt controls on the Internet, as happens in China), and scholars worry about the way that the Internet facilitates the spread of AIDS denialism.[57] The *Medical Hypotheses* saga was not about silencing Duesberg, but rather an attempt to ensure that his work is subject to some meaningful editorial review if it is to bear the imprimatur of science.

8

THE CONSPIRATORIAL MOVE
AND THE STRUGGLE FOR
EVIDENCE-BASED MEDICINE

E arlier chapters argued that AIDS denialism and AIDS origin conspiracy theories both make a conspiratorial move against HIV science. Not only does this undermine HIV-prevention messages, but it leaves people vulnerable to exploitation by cultropreneurs offering untested alternative remedies in the place of antiretrovirals. What makes AIDS denialism particularly worrying is that it has a strong social basis constructed around the roles of hero scientist, living icon, cultropreneur, and praise-singer—all of which assist in forging new forms of identity and social solidarity in opposition to biomedicine. But precisely because these roles are important, they present targets for HIV scientists and AIDS activists in the struggle against them.

Such roles and contestation are not unique to AIDS. For example, the anti-vaccination movement that sprang up around the "hero scientist" Andrew Wakefield was also replete with praise-singers, cultropreneurs, and living icons. And, like the Duesberg case, criticisms were made by scientists against the journal that published Wakefield's research. This concluding chapter points to the similarities between the two cases—especially with regard to the way conspiracy theories are evoked to construct credibility and deflect criticism—and locates both within the broader defense of evidence-based medicine.

THE MMR SCARE: ECHOES WITH AIDS DENIALISM

In 1998 the *Lancet* published a paper by Andrew Wakefield and others from the London Royal Free Hospital suggesting a link between the mumps, measles, and rubella (MMR) vaccine and autism.[1] Based on a case series of twelve children with intestinal and mental developmental disorders, the paper reported that parents of eight of the nine autistic children had associated the onset of autism with the MMR vaccine. Wakefield highlighted those parental fears at a press conference and, going beyond the conclusions of the paper, suggested that the MMR vaccine may well have damaged the guts of these children, thereby supposedly allowing harmful proteins to enter the bloodstream and damage the brain.[2] Although only one in five children in his study developed bowel problems before they manifested developmental disorders (hence such cause and effect was unlikely), Wakefield told reporters that there was "sufficient concern" in his own mind "for a case to be made for vaccines to be given individually at not less than one-year intervals."[3]

Wakefield claimed it was a "moral issue" for him and that he could not support the triple MMR vaccine until his concerns had been resolved. But as he had patented a single-dose vaccine for measles a year earlier, he stood to benefit directly from a swing away from the MMR vaccine. He failed to disclose this, or that he was receiving payments from a lawyer planning to sue manufacturers of the MMR vaccine, or that the parents of some of the children in his study were involved in the legal action (which meant the selection into his study was seriously biased). These ethical problems, as well as his failure to obtain ethical clearance for the research and his subjecting the children to invasive and unnecessary procedures, resulted in the British Medical Council subsequently finding him guilty of misconduct and in the *Lancet* withdrawing the paper.[4] Nonetheless, in the interim Wakefield's paper and related publicity generated a major backlash against the MMR vaccine in the UK.

Like Duesberg, Wakefield made good use of the media to create skepticism toward mainstream science and to suggest that a genuine scientific debate was being oppressed. He accused the UK's Department of Health of relegating "scientific issues to the bottom of the barrel in favor of winning a propaganda war."[5] In 2000 he took his battle to the United States, testifying in congressional hearings on the vaccine-autism link and appearing on the television program *60 Minutes* to advise against the use of the triple vaccine.[6] The following year, he moved to the United States, saying that the hostility toward him in England had become untenable. Echoing Mbeki's objectification of the scientific community as part of a systemic "omnipotent apparatus," he told journalists: "I realise now that everything that has happened to me was inevitable from the beginning. If you offend the system, then the system will take its revenge."[7] The media picked up the hint of conspiracy, and two years later a conspiratorial docudrama was aired on British television lionizing Wakefield and the parents of autistic children who support him—while suggesting that government officials had been plotting against him, stealing his files, tapping his phone, and so on.[8]

As with Duesberg's case, Wakefield's praise-singers contributed to his scientist-oppressed-by-the-establishment image. Journalist Justine Picardie reported on the "dark tales" she had heard about bugging devices and stolen records, and asked in a discourse laden with suspicion why "his supporters in the medical establishment fear speaking out openly on the issue," and why "so many parents of autistic children believe there has been a concerted cover-up of evidence suggesting a possible link between the vaccine and their children's condition." She observed that the conspiracy theories circulating around Wakefield may perhaps be no more than the "overheated product of too many viewings of Hollywood films," but then added: "It's not hard to imagine Russell Crowe playing Dr. Wakefield, opposite Julia Roberts as a feisty single mother fighting for justice for her child."[9] Melanie Phillips of London's *Daily Mail* similarly represented him as a hero long after his theory that MMR caused autism had been disproved,[10] and Lorraine Fraser of the *Telegraph* wrote a series of articles heroizing him for defying the "official wisdom" and "risking the wrath" of the US Department of Health.[11] Neither questioned his evidence or seriously inquired as to why the medical establishment condemned him.

A systematic review of the media coverage of MMR and its impact on public opinion concluded that mainstream medical science came off second best, in large part because the parents with their autistic children assumed the role of living icons:

> many media reports gave voice to both sides in the ensuing debate about the safety of the vaccine. This was sometimes a debate between scientists and sometimes a debate between scientists or public health officials and concerned parents. The role of parents in this balancing act allowed anecdotal evidence from parents with autistic children to enter the discussion—which, while not authoritative as scientific evidence, is powerful rhetorically. Indeed scientists or public health officials cannot have relished debating people who not only command immediate public sympathy, but whose own children were, apparently, testimony to the risks involved with vaccination.[12]

Sensationalist coverage of the MMR story reached its height when Britain's then prime minister, Tony Blair, refused to answer the question whether his young son, Leo, had had the triple vaccine. Given the widely reported New Age predilections of Blair's wife, Cheri, it was all too easy for people to believe that Leo had not had the MMR vaccine. For example, Sylvia Caplin, who reportedly conducted "channeling" for Cheri Blair,[13] condemned the "toxic" MMR vaccine for being "too much, too soon and in the wrong formula,"[14] and Jack Temple, the Blair's "douser and homeopathic healer" openly promoted an "energy-giving homeopathic alternative remedy" that supposedly eliminated the need for all vaccines.[15]

According to the media evaluation and impact study cited above, the importance of Blair's position as prime minister was crucial:

> For people confused about who to trust, this was an important indicator of the government's faith in its own position. In a nutshell, was the government's support for MMR deeply felt or merely tactical or strategic? Leo Blair might, therefore, be reasonably seen as a test of the government's confidence in its own position. . . . If Leo Blair *had* been given the MMR vaccine, our findings suggest that the Prime Minister's refusal to disclose this information (while understandable on a personal level) was, in public health terms, a mistake. It kept open the possibility that the Prime Minister had

reviewed the evidence and decided against the MMR jab, which can only
have added to people's fears.[16]

Although this episode of poor leadership is but a pale reflection of the
mistakes made by President Mbeki, it stands as a further example of how
leaders can undermine public health by raising, or even appearing to raise,
doubts about mainstream science. Coverage of the Leo Blair story peaked
in 2002. During this time, opinion polls reported that only about half of
respondents said they would vaccinate their child with MMR.[17] The pro-
portion of children receiving the MMR vaccine dropped from over 90 percent to 70 percent and, in some areas of London, to 50 percent.[18] Although
uptake subsequently increased to 85 percent in 2010, this remains below the
92 percent level achieved before the MMR scare—and below that required
for community immunity. Measles cases continue to rise.[19]

As was the case with AIDS denialism, many physicians and scientists
were alarmed and angry—both by the quality of Wakefield's work and his
impact on vaccination rates. Immediately after the publication of Wakefield's paper, the *Lancet* was flooded with letters from doctors, scientists,
and public health officials angry that the journal had published such a potentially incendiary paper based on a very small number of cases. But the
editor, Roger Horton, was unrepentant, retorting that there "is an unpleas-
ant whiff of arrogance in this whole debate" and asking rhetorically, "can
the public not be trusted with a controversial hypothesis?"[20]

There are some echoes here with the *Medical Hypotheses* saga, although
in this case the issue was whether the paper had been reviewed adequately
rather than whether it had been reviewed at all. Paul Offit, a pediatrician
and vaccine scientist, criticized Horton for "ignoring the criticisms of several reviewers" and for "not anticipating the public reaction."[21] Other commentators were less restrained. Henry Miller, a molecular biologist and former official at the NIH and FDA accused Horton of making a "mockery
of the peer review and publication process." When Wakefield's article was
finally withdrawn in 2010, Miller editorialized on *Forbes*:

> The Wakefield article caused incalculable damage by eliciting public skepti-
> cism about the safety of vaccines, which has caused plummeting vaccina-
> tion rates in Europe and the US and a resurgence of cases of infectious

diseases that had become rare. Richard Horton, editor of *The Lancet*, denied any culpability, whining that Wakefield "deceived the journal." Bollocks. A groundbreaking study that appears to be implausible and turns popular medical wisdom on its head needs to be done on more than 12 patients and an examination of the actual patient records.[22]

Horton argued that until Wakefield had been found guilty of misconduct twelve years later, he had no proof that Wakefield's 1998 paper was deceptive.[23] However, back in 2004, Brian Deer, an investigative journalist for the London *Sunday Times*, had told him about Wakefield's conflict of interest issues involving at least five of the children in his study and that Wakefield had never received ethical clearance for the study.[24] When this became known, ten of Wakefield's twelve coauthors disassociated themselves from the paper. Yet the *Lancet* declined to withdraw the paper, even as further evidence accumulated showing no causal link between vaccines and autism[25] and against Wakefield's hypothesis that vaccines cause leaky guts and chronic infections.[26]

In the meantime, the paper lent legitimacy to those opposing the MMR vaccine and promoting alternative theories, some of them harmful treatments such as chelation therapy, testosterone ablation, and electric shock.[27] Jenny McCarthy, the celebrity "activist mom" of the US vaccines-cause-autism movement, claims to have cured her son of autism[28] and advises parents to ignore the negative messages from medical science and to "try everything"[29] in their search for a cure. She heads an enterprise called Generation Rescue, which *inter alia* promotes her three best-selling books, and remains a strong supporter of Wakefield. When he was convicted of misconduct, she released a press statement saying that he had been tried by a "kangaroo court where public health officials in the pocket of vaccine makers served as judge and jury" and that he and parents of autistic children were being "subjected to a remarkable media campaign engineered by vaccine manufacturers."[30] Her use of the conspiracy trope to defend Wakefield is almost identical to that employed by AIDS denialists to defend Duesberg.

Wakefield refused to concede any wrong-doing. At the time of writing, he was still executive director of Thoughtful House, an American center for treatment and research on autistic children which contests the scientific consensus on vaccine safety, insists that the idea that vaccines cause autism is still "on the table," and promotes the use of single vaccines rather than combination vaccines like MMR.[31] The key service appears to be colonoscopies, but in a discourse reminiscent of that of cultropreneurs, the center also provides "holistic" treatments for autistic children, including supporting so-called "detoxification pathways."[32]

In sum, the role of dissident "hero scientist" is clearly symbolically important for the AIDS denialist and anti-vaccination movements. Precisely because the label "scientific" lends credibility to their claims, both Duesberg and Wakefield sought to publish in the "scientific" stable of journals. In the case of Duesberg, boundary work by HIV scientists and others resulted in the withdrawal of one of his papers and in the editorial policy of the journal being changed. In the case of Wakefield, the boundary work was slower and more institutionalized, but the result was more decisive: withdrawal of his paper and his disbarment from medical practice in the UK. In both cases, the papers were stripped of any imprimatur of science they once had—and in both cases their supporters blamed this on a corrupt and bullying scientific establishment. Yet they maintain a degree of social legitimacy, in part through the conspiratorial moves employed by their supporters to justify their marginalization, and in part because of broader public skepticism toward medical science and tolerance for alternative healing modalities. It is to this phenomenon—and the way that pro-science activists are increasingly challenging it—that we now turn.

MEDICAL MISTRUST AND ALTERNATIVE MEDICINE

The rise in popularity and respectability of alternative medicine is reflected in the evolution of popular discourse about it. What was once dubbed "pseudoscience," "chicanery," and "quackery" is now typically referred to as "alternative and complementary" or "holistic" therapy. Even the term *health* is making way in some contexts for *wellness*, partly to incorporate the number of non-biomedical and unproven interventions which are now accepted by many as a necessary part of healing. Remedies and healing modalities that used to circulate on the countercultural fringe have become so widely used that they are now accepted as mainstream. This has blurred the boundaries between what used to be the "stigmatized knowledge domain" of the cultic milieu and conventional medical practice. It has also made boundary work in defense of evidence-based medicine increasingly challenging.

One of the reasons for public suspicion toward medical science has to do with the fact that a great deal of medical research is conducted in the private sector, where profitability and the drive for patentable drugs take center stage. Pharmaceutical companies have been known to provide incentives to doctors to encourage certain prescription practices, to abuse the patent law to prevent lower-cost competition, and to devote excessive resources toward developing and marketing "me too" drugs rather than searching for genuinely innovative interventions.[33] They have also been known to bias the results of clinical trials—for example, testing a drug against inadequate doses of a competitor, using multiple end points and then selecting the ones that suit the desired outcomes best, presenting subgroup analyses when they produce desired results, and so on.[34] Most notoriously, in the Vioxx trial, Merck researchers shortened the reporting period for adverse effects—notably heart attacks—but not for other outcomes and side effects for which Vioxx performed relatively well.[35] When the Lancet published a meta-analysis showing that the unacceptable risks of Vioxx had been evident four years before the drug was withdrawn,[36] an accompanying editorial castigated Merck and the regulators for acting out of "ruthless, short-sighted and irresponsible self-interest."[37] Understandably, such highly publicized events promote skepticism toward the pharmaceutical industry and fuels fears that biomedical drugs have not been properly tested and may actually cause serious harm.

There is clearly a range of serious issues here, which is why calls have been made for greater regulation of the marketing practices of pharmaceutical companies, for the publication of a clinical trial register, and greater transparency with regard to the conduct of clinical trials, analysis of data, and presentation of results.[38] The key point, though, is that these problems do not warrant what science journalist Jon Cohen calls "pharmanoia," i.e., that suspicious stance which "puts Big Pharma on a par with Big Tobacco" and turns "shades of moral grey into black."[39] And it certainly does not justify the linked embrace of unscientific propositions. As Ben Goldacre complains, "'Big Pharma is evil' goes the line of reasoning, 'therefore homeopathy works and the MMR vaccine causes autism.'This is probably not helpful."[40]

MODERN FORMS OF BOUNDARY WORK IN DEFENSE OF SCIENCE

Because the rejection of medical science has adverse implications for public health—as evidenced by unnecessary AIDS deaths and declining vaccination rates—this cultural tolerance for alternative medicine has not gone unchallenged, especially in the Internet era. In the past, those wishing to explore the cultic milieu and related alternative lifestyles did so primarily by subscribing to print editions of alternative healing magazines such as *Mothering*—the magazine that featured a cover photograph of Christine Maggiore with "No AZT" emblazoned on her pregnant abdomen. Today, like many other fringe publications, *Mothering* no longer produces a print edition. Consumers of alternative health services now surf the Internet like everyone else. In so doing, they will encounter alternative websites by the dozen, but they will also come across anti–AIDS denial sites and advice from conventional medical practitioners. They will find sites telling them Maggiore's daughter Eliza Jane died because a doctor gave her an antibiotic and that Maggiore died of stress—but they will also find information showing that both Eliza Jane and Maggiore died of AIDS. The Internet, in other words, is both a source of opportunity for cultropreneurs—and a site of danger for them as converts can easily be lost.

This determination to fight back and expose the dangers of denialism is evident also in the more conventional print media. For example, the popular magazine for science and reason, *Skeptical Inquirer*, which started off life investigating claims about UFO sightings, ghosts, psychic powers, and similar paranormal phenomena gradually found its focus shifting increasingly to exposing the claims of alternative healers.[41] More recently, medical professionals such as Goldacre, Kalichman, and Offit have penned popular books critiquing bad science, AIDS denialism, and the anti-vaccination movement.[42] As such, they form part of a broader critical set of writings about the false claims and dangers of alternative medicine—for example, Dan Hurley's exposé of the US vitamin and herbal supplement industry, Edzard Ernst and Simon Singh's evaluation of the evidence for alternative therapies, and Michael Specter's critique of denialism and irrational thinking.[43] It is too early to tell whether this counteroffensive by pro-science advocates has achieved much success, but the fact that Goldacre and Singh have both been sued for libel (unsuccessfully) by alternative therapists suggests that some of their blows have hit home.[44]

The electronic media has proved to be a crucial mobilizing instrument for pro-science activists. Supporters of Simon Singh used Twitter and Facebook to keep abreast of the libel case, to organize events, and to lobby for reform of the UK's libel laws. Both Goldacre and Kalichman operate blogs on topics linked to their books, and they are active within the broader community of pro-science Internet activists.[45] Goldacre refers to the wider group of pro-science bloggers as "the posse" and posts links to them on his website.[46] And their actions are not merely intellectual. When the British Chiropractic Association sued Singh, the posse flooded the association with complaints about individual chiropractors, all of which required investigation. For Goldacre, the lessons are clear:

> First, if you have reputation and superficial plausibility more than evidence to support your activities, then it may be wise to keep under the radar, rather than start expensive fights. But more interestingly than that, a ragged band of bloggers from all walks of life has, to my mind, done a better job of subjecting an entire industry's claims to meaningful, public, scientific scrutiny than the media, the industry itself, and even its own regulator. It's strange this task has fallen to them, but I'm glad someone is doing it, and they do it very, very well indeed.[47]

In other words, boundary work in defense of science has not only adapted to the modern age by taking place online and with the help of electronic media, but it is being undertaken by members of the public. Whereas, in the past, boundary work was conducted primarily by scholars seeking to develop and maintain public respect for science and to relegate "pseudosciences" like phrenology[48] beyond the pale of academia, today the battle is more diffuse, public, and decentralized—indeed often fought at an individual level via cut-and-thrust debate on blog postings. As Goldacre suggests, it may be that this is more effective than action taken by the scientific community.

Damien Thompson is similarly optimistic, noting in his populist polemic *Counterknowledge: How We Surrendered to Conspiracy Theories, Quack Medicine, Bogus Science and Fake History* that high-profile alternative therapists have proved "surprisingly vulnerable to guerrilla attacks from the blogosphere":

> Freelance defenders of empirical truth, armed to the teeth with hard data, have mounted devastating ambushes on quacks and frauds who have ventured too far into the public domain. The tactic is an antiretroviral rather than a vaccine, and too modest in scope to effect dramatic change in society, but it does seem to work. . . . Reputations are easily damaged in a furiously competitive market, and people rather enjoy the spectacle of smug, rich lifestyle gurus being humiliated.[49]

This social phenomenon of "angry nerds" and "guerilla bloggers" dedicated to defending evidence-based medicine and challenging quackery is important. Rather than relying on the scientific community to defend the boundaries of science, we are seeing a much more socially embedded struggle over values and how we should be approaching our health and that of others.

WILL THIS POPULAR ENLIGHTENMENT PROJECT WORK?

Defending science is a quintessentially enlightenment project. It assumes that progress is possible through reason and the accumulation of evidence, and that the scientific method is persuasive and can be made more so. Those who engage in the defense of science necessarily reject relativist approaches to the truth as unreasonable, defeatist, and dangerous. Thompson is particularly dismissive of those who have "turned their backs on the methodology that enables us to distinguish fact from fantasy" and concludes that it "will be their fault if the sleep of reason brings forth monsters."[50] Goldacre is similarly critical of "humanities graduates" for wearing their ignorance of science as a "badge of honour" while viewing scientists as "socially powerful, arbitrary, unelected authority figures."[51] In his view, this has had demonstrably adverse effects on public health because of the lack of trust in, or appreciation of, the evidence-based medicine it promotes.

Reasserting the enlightenment project of progress through reason and evidence is one thing. But whether such progress is possible remains an open question. How easy is it to persuade people through factual corrections of their misperceptions? The answer seems to depend a great deal on the individual. For example, AIDS denialists like Maggiore are impervious to corrective evidence about HIV science because they are, as Kalichman observes, in a psychological state of encapsulated delusion (chapter 6). They are impossible to argue with, and indeed it may even be counterproductive to do so. According to recent research in political psychology, providing people who are ideologically committed to a particular view with "preference-incongruent information" can "backfire" by causing them to support their original argument even more strongly.[52] This could be because they misread or reinterpret the information to support their original position, or because they "counterargue" the information in their minds, thereby increasing their intellectual commitment to it.

The problem is, in part, a general one. Summarizing a substantial body of psychological literature, Brendan Nyhan and Jason Reifler note that humans are "goal-directed information processors who tend to evaluate information with a directional bias towards reinforcing their pre-existing views."[53] Farhad Manjoo, for similar reasons, worries that our tendency for "selective exposure" is resulting in reality "splitting" as we "choose our personal versions of truth by subscribing to the clutch of specialists we find agreeable and trustworthy."[54] He argues that the digital revolution has exacerbated the problem because now you can watch, listen to and read what you want, whenever you want; seek out and discuss, in exhaustive and insular detail, the kind of news that pleases you; and indulge your political, social or scientific theories, whether sophisticated or naïve, extremist or banal, grounded in reality or so far out you're floating in an asteroid belt, among people who feel exactly the same way.[55]

Jodi Dean takes the argument even further, claiming that the Internet destroys "the illusion of the public by creating innumerable networks of connection and information," which negates "any possibility of agreement" because "consensus reality" no longer exists.[56] She argues that we cannot judge the rationality of people who believe they have been abducted by aliens and that we no longer have "widespread criteria for judgments about what is reasonable and what is not."[57]

But while Manjoo and Dean are highlighting the ways in which the electronic media facilitates the growth of rival thought communities, their pessimism about the enlightenment project goes too far. As Michael Barkun points out, the boundary between mainstream and stigmatized knowledge domains may have become more "permeable," but the world has yet to enter a state of "complete epistemological pluralism."[58] The fact that Duesberg and Wakefield keep trying to get the imprimatur of science for their discredited ideas speaks to the ongoing public prestige and power of science. Furthermore, their support base is far from fixed in stone. Whereas some people have become so committed to their unorthodox views that they cannot be moved from them—such as the hero scientists and living icons of the AIDS denialist and anti-vaccine movements—this is the exception rather than the rule for people dabbling in the cultic milieu. The cultic milieu may well be an oppositional subculture inherently suspicious of scientific practice and tolerant of mysticism and conspiracy theories, yet reason and judgment are not abandoned by all who enter it.

Indeed, as indicated by the correspondent on Kalichman's blog (chapter 6) who described how Maggiore's death from pneumonia started the process of getting him thinking that maybe he had been wrong in rejecting HIV science, people motivated to explore the cultic milieu are open to changing their minds. And, as the focus group of AIDS origin conspiracy believers in Cape Town (chapter 2) also illustrated, seemingly strong endorsements of oppositional beliefs turn out to be more fluid and contingent when openly discussed. Similarly, the comments by prisoners about David Gilbert's critique of AIDS conspiracy theory show that politically sensitive arguments that both acknowledge the reasonable basis for conspiracy beliefs while seeking also to correct them can result in people changing their minds (chapter 4).

To return to Colin Campbell's seminal work on the cultic milieu, he stresses that this is not a cultural space where firm opinions are held, but it is rather a "society of seekers":

> Seekership is probably the one characteristic that all members of cultic groups have in common, and while this facilitates the formation of groups, it poses special problems for their maintenance. Seekers do not necessarily cease seeking when a revealed truth is offered to them, nor do they necessarily stop looking in other directions when one path is indicated as the path to the truth.[59]

This, in turn, creates the space for pro-science activists to compete for the attention of those seeking information about health and healing. By doing this in the electronic world, through dedicated websites and blogs, and by posting comments in response to claims by cultropreneurs, the Internet becomes a tougher place for people to sequestrate themselves in a comfortable cocoon of the like-minded. These days, a "google search," the modern-day equivalent of practical seekership, catapults one from AIDS denialist to pro-science activist websites, and exposes a person to news (like Maggiore's death) which sites like Alive and Well prefer to downplay, if not hide.

This is good news for the enlightenment project. As Nyhan and Reifler note in their review of the psychological literature, people may be biased in favor of interpretations that align with their prior prejudices and suppositions—but this does not mean that they just believe what they like and never accept counter-attitudinal information. Nyhan and Reifler cite early studies showing that when faced with "information of sufficient quantity or clarity," people do change their minds,[60] and their own research backs this up.[61]

The challenge for the pro-science advocacy movement is thus to keep an active and credible presence on the Internet, both with regard to exposing the cultropreneurs and promoting evidence-based medicine. In so doing, they need to educate people about the power of science while also acknowledging that scientific practice is contested, socially structured, and can be biased and shoddy (as Merck's Vioxx study and Wakefield's research illustrates). Recognizing and exposing the limitations of science not only builds credibility by acknowledging reasonable concerns, but assists the broader project of promoting good science.

The Internet is an anarchic space where popular forms of boundary work in defense of science range from ridicule and banter to serious discussion about scientific findings along with URLs to scientific articles and reports. It looks, in other words, like the varied countercultural, seeking space that used to be the preserve only of the cultic milieu—but with greater informational depth. The weapons of science and reason are still very much in contention, both within the scientific community and in this creative popular space.

NOTES

1. THE CONSPIRATORIAL MOVE AGAINST HIV SCIENCE AND ITS CONSEQUENCES

1. Lapidos (2008). See also Kincaid (2008) on white right-winger and AIDS conspiracy theorist Leonard Horowitz's influence on Jeremiah Wright.
2. "Nobel Winner: AIDS a WMD"; see www.news24.com/Africa/News/Nobel-winner-Aids-a-WMD-20041009.
3. See Bogart and Bird (2003), Bogart and Thorburn (2005), Ross, Essien, and Torres (2006), and Bogart, Galvan et al. (2010) for the United States, and Grebe and Nattrass (2011) for South Africa.
4. Bogart, Wagner et al. (2010).
5. See Bohnert and Latkin (2009) for the United States, and Bogart, Wagner et al. (2010) and Tun et al. (2010) for South Africa. Also, in the Cape Area Panel Study, the odds of having ever been tested for HIV are significantly lower for respondents who endorse AIDS origin conspiracy beliefs (odds ratio: 0.58, 95%; confidence interval: 0.44–0.77).
6. These cases are discussed in chapters 2 and 8, respectively.
7. See, for example, Keeley (1999, 2003), Räikkä (2009), and Basham (2003) for a discussion of the philosophical reasons why one cannot reject conspiracy theory on any *a priori* basis.

8. Keeley (2003:106).
9. Keeley (1999:126).
10. Campbell (2002).
11. Frazier (2009).

2. AIDS ORIGIN CONSPIRACY THEORIES IN THE UNITED STATES AND SOUTH AFRICA

1. DeParle (1990).
2. Crocker et al. (1999), Goertzel (1994), Ross, Essien, and Torres (2006), and Darrow, Montanea, and Gladwin (2009).
3. Hutchinson et al. (2007:604), and Clark et al. (2008).
4. Almost 30% of respondents recruited in clinics for sexually transmitted infections believed AIDS was introduced by white people to control black Africans (Bogart, Kalichman, and Simbayi 2010); 25% of a sample of African gay men in Pretoria believed that HIV was invented in a laboratory (Tun et al. 2010); and 51.4% of a sample of AIDS patients in the Northern Province thought that AIDS had or may have been "invented by whites to kill blacks" (Navario 2009:172).
5. Campsmith et al. (2008).
6. Briggs (2004).
7. Rubincam (2008).
8. See, for example, Sabatier (1988), Chirimuuta and Chirumuuta (1989), Turner (1994), Farmer (1993), Treichler (1999), Rödlach (2006), and Butt (2005).
9. Treichler (1999:220).
10. Cochrane (1987), Fine (1992).
11. Fine (1992:55).
12. Rödlach (2006).
13. Goldstuck (1990:155).
14. Niehaus and Jonsson (2005).
15. Finnegan (2001), Berger and Gould (2002).
16. Berger and Gould (2002:1).
17. Ibid., 7.
18. Willsher (1999). Note that with the exception of injections and deliberate sexual infection, all of these putative pathways are biologically implausible.
19. Ibid.
20. Niehaus and Jonsson (2005:197–98).
21. Ashforth (2002:124).
22. Willsher (1999).
23. See, for example, Henderson (2005:40–41), Posel, Kahn, and Waker (2007:7–8), and Niehaus and Jonsson (2005:195–96).

24. Henderson (2005) and Steinberg (2008:138).
25. Nattrass (1994).
26. The focus groups were run in Xhosa by Thobani Ncaphayi on August 11, 2010, and transcribed and translated by Unathi Kondile. The research process was designed and led by Clara Rubincam, with the assistance of Nicoli Nattrass and Eduard Grebe, for the AIDS and Society Research Unit, University of Cape Town (UCT).
27. Steinberg (2008:146–47).
28. Farmer (1993:227).
29. Hofstadter (1965).
30. Ibid., 29.
31. Barrell (2000).
32. Geffen and Cameron (2009:1–2).
33. Kirk (2000).
34. See Cooper (1991) and www.remnantradio.org/Archives/articles/William%20Cooper/Behold.A.Pale.Horse%202.mp3. For a discussion of conspiracy theories about the Illuminati and the fraudulent claims they are based upon, see Aaronovitch (2009).
35. Barkun (2003:181).
36. Ibid., 60.
37. These are available at www.remnantradio.org/Archives/articles/William%20Cooper/WC.htm.
38. Barkun (2003:95).
39. Shaffer (2001_.
40. See www.remnantradio.org/Archives/articles/William%20Cooper/WC.htm.
41. Shaffer (2001).
42. Kirk (2000).
43. Although Horowitz is best known for his alternative healing business, he has also been described as "the right's most visible authority on medical matters" (Barkun 2003:162).
44. The Nation of Islam's publication *Final Call* has run positive articles on Horowitz and his AIDS conspiracy tract (Horowitz 1996), including posting links to his website. Horowitz, in turn, heaps praises on Farrakhan for his views on medical genocide and for speaking out against the "medical cartel" (Shabazz 2004). See also the interview with Horowitz by Saltan Muhammad (Jan. 29, 2003) in www.finalcall.com/artman/publish/Perspectives_1/AIDS_The_greatest_weapon_of_mass_destruction_439.shtml.
45. Lapidos (2008). See also Kincaid (2008) on Horowitz's influence on Jeremiah Wright.
46. Links to his books and summaries of his key claims are available through his website; see www.tetrahedron.org.

47. See www.healthyworldstore.com.

48. See www.healthyworldaffiliates.com/oxysilver-c-82.html.

49. See www.healthyworldaffiliates.com/oxysilver-c-82.html (accessed Oct. 29, 2010).

50. The letter from the FDA to Horowitz is available at www.fda.gov/ICECI/EnforcementActions/WarningLetters/ucm212397.htm.

51. See, for example, Bertlet (2009:30), who highlights shared anti-Semitism, and Gardell (2002), who points to shared opposition to universalism between black and white separatists.

52. Campbell (2002:14).

53. When he first identified the cultic milieu as a social phenomenon in the early 1970s, Campbell identified "the religious tradition of mysticism and the personal service practices of healing and divination" as its two key elements. More recently, others have argued that the cultic milieu has broadened to include a wider range of oppositional activities, including the green movement, anti-globalization protestors, right-wing militia members, etc., and that far from being the fringe oppositional counterculture it was in the early 1970s, many of its practices, especially with regard to alternative medicine, have emerged to challenge the dominant culture, e.g. Kaplan and Lööw (2002:1–2) and Gardell (2002).

54. Hofstadter (1965:7).

55. Kelly (1995:62).

56. Ibid., 64.

57. Bertlet (2009:16).

58. See Sabatier (1988:66), Chirimuuta and Chirumuuta (1989), Farmer (1993), and Rödlach (2006).

59. US Department of State (1987:10).

60. Andrew and Gordievsky (1990) and Koehler (1999:260–61).

61. US Department of State (1987:2–3).

62. This is not an altogether preposterous idea given recent revelations about how Guatemalan prisoners and inmates of mental hospitals were used in syphilis treatment experiments by researchers from the US Public Health Service, the National Institutes of Health, and the Guatemalan government between 1946 and 1948 (Reverby 2011).

63. US Department of State (1987:5–7).

64. Andrew and Gordievsky (1990), Sabatier (1988:64–66), US Department of State (1987:12).

65. Whitfield (2000b) and Gilbert (2004a).

66. US Department of State (1987:10).

67. Andrew and Gordievsky (1990:631).

68. Hitchens (1993:14).

69. See discussion in Chirimuuta and Chirimuuta (1989).

70. Curtis (1992), Kyle (1992), and Elswood and Stricker (1994).

71. Hooper (2000).

72. Cohen (2000a) and Offit (2008:112–13).

73. Cohen (2000b).

74. Plotkin, quoted in ibid., 1850.

75. Cohen (2000a).

76. Hooper (2003).

77. See, for example, Martin (2010).

78. Worobey et al. (2004) and Sharp and Hahn (2010:2489).

79. Van Heuverswyn and Peeters (2007).

80. Korber et al. (2000) and Worobey et al. (2008).

81. Iliffe (2006)

82. Chitnis, Rawls, and Moore (2000) and Moore (2004).

83. Harris and Paxman (1982:103–135).

84. Ibid., 168.

85. Ibid., 166.

86. Ibid., 158–59.

87. Ibid., 160–68.

88. Hatch (2003:19).

89. Ibid., 24.

90. See www.youtube.com/watch?v=CDxZ7PX8YGI.

91. The first reference was to Herrera, Adamson, and Gallo (1970), demonstrating that uptake of transfer ribonucleic acid was possible *in vitro* in normal and leukemic cells. Gallo pointed out that this was research conducted in the 1960s, long before genetic cloning had been invented and before he started working in virology. The second reference was to a published paper reporting the presence of reverse transcriptase in cells from a lymphoma patient and noting that similar links with cancer were evident in other mammals (Gallo et al. 1971). Despite the dramatic overlays on the video and strong suggestions by Horowitz that this was the crucial smoking gun, the paper has absolutely nothing to do with combining viruses and creating new ones.

92. Harris and Paxman (1982:266).

93. US Congress, House of Representatives, *U.S. Department of Defense Appropriations for 1970: Hearings before a Subcommittee of the Committee on Appropriations*, 91st Cong., 1st sess., July 1, 1969; chairman, George H. Mahon (D-TX).

94. Graves (2001:6).

95. Ibid., 29.

96. Johnson (1985:49).

97. Ibid., 73.
98. Marcus (1999:3–4).
99. Johnson (1985:57).
100. Ibid., 73. The KGB probably used such a device to inject Georgi Markov (a Bulgarian dissident writer) with a lethal dose of ricin poison in London in 1978.
101. Whitfield (2000b:n.p.).
102. Graves (2001:12–13); see also www.boydgraves.com/timeline/.
103. Horowitz's website (www.tetrahedron.org) advertises his books and documentaries and sells various of his "alternative" cures and remedies. Updated summaries of his views on the origin of AIDS can be found at http://tetra hedron.org/articles/aids-coverups/aids_coverups.html and www.originofaids .com/articles/early.htm.
104. See, for example, Cantwell (1988, 1993) and an interview with Cantwell at www.rense.com/general74/cantww.htm.
105. Graves (2001:26).
106. See www.boydgraves.com/flowchart/ or http://images.biafranigeriaworld .com/BNW-1971-AIDS-Flowchart-Full-Size.jpg.
107. Graves (2001:10, 32).
108. Ibid.
109. See www.devvy.com/aids_20001206.html.
110. He petitioned Rep. Stephanie Tubbs Jones, the first black woman to represent Ohio in Congress, and Rep. James Traficant (both D-OH), who then asked the US General Accounting Office to investigate Graves's claims. Their reply, and the associated report detailing Graves's legal outcomes and summarizing expert opinion and key facts, is available at www.gao.gov/new.items/d02809r .pdf.
111. See interview with Boyd Graves in *The Final Call*, Oct. 5, 2004; see www.final call.com/artman/publish/Perspectives_1/AIDS_is_man-made_-Interview_ with_Dr_Boyd_Graves_1597.shtml.
112. A summary of his claims is available at www.rense.com/general20/rabb.htm.
113. See www.rexresearch.com/antelman/silverox.htm.
114. For detailed information about the claims made by Antelman and the connection to Boyd Graves, see www.scribd.com/doc/29091515/Understanding-Tetrasil-Ag4O4-the-AIDS-cure-patent-and-dosage-progress-diary. According to this blog post, Antelman sent an e-mail claiming that trials had been run in South Africa, but there is no way to confirm this; see www.abovetop secret.com/forum/thread200422/pg1.
115. See www.thebody.com/Forums/AIDS/Meds/Archive/Alternative/Q154827 .html.

116. See interview with Boyd Graves in *The Final Call*, Oct. 5, 2004; see note 111 and http://bodygraves.blogspot.com/. That he promoted the cure in Zambia has been confirmed by AIDS activists (private correspondence).
117. Interview with Boyd Graves in *Final Call*, Oct. 5, 2004.
118. Pipes (1997:5–6), Whitfield (2000b), and Bertlet (2009:35).
119. Gilbert (2004a).
120. Blackstock (1976) and Chomsky (1976).
121. Berger (2006:63–64).
122. See, for example, Blackstock (1976:92).
123. Johnson (1985:223–24).
124. Price (2007a, 2007b).
125. Harris and Paxman (1982:206).
126. Thomas and Quinn (1991) and Reverby (2009).
127. Dalton (1989:221).
128. These articles are available at www.maga.nu:8080/ampp/webb.html.
129. Pipes (1997:4–5).
130. Hellinger (2003:215).
131. Whitfield (2000b).
132. Quoted in ibid.
133. Katz et al. (2008).
134. Gamble (1997).
135. Brandon, Isaac, and LaVeist (2005).

3. WHO BELIEVES AIDS CONSPIRACY THEORIES AND WHY LEADERSHIP MATTERS

1. Niehaus and Jonsson (2005:195).
2. Ibid., 202.
3. Bogart and Thorburn (2006:1145).
4. Parsons et al. (1999:217).
5. Klonoff and Landrine (1999:456).
6. Gwata (2009).
7. Hofstadter (1965:3–4).
8. Showalter 1997: 5, 12.
9. Kessler et al. (2002) and Strine et al. (2005).
10. Strine et al. (2005:1134).
11. Hofstadter (1965:38–43).
12. See Jameson (1991) and the discussion in Mason (2002:40).
13. See, for example, Knight (2002), Willman (2002), and Mason (2002).

14. Dean (1998:144).
15. See, for example, Knight (2002:9), Thomas and Quinn (1993:133–34), and Goertzel (1994:739).
16. Lyotard (1984).
17. Appadurai (1996).
18. Treichler (1999:15).
19. See, for example, Hellinger (2003) and Bratich (2008), who argues that depending on how they are articulated, conspiracy theories could complement political concerns and act as a catalyst to new forms of analysis and action (119).
20. Melley (2002:63).
21. Mirowsky and Ross (1983:238).
22. Goertzel (1994).
23. Abalakina-Paap and Stephan (1999).
24. See, for example, Crocker et al. (1999:949).
25. Evans-Pritchard (1937).
26. Wilson (1951), Comaroff and Comaroff (1993, 2002), Geschiere (1997).
27. Sanders and West (2003:6–7).
28. See Stadler (2003), Kalichman and Simbayi (2004), Ashforth (2002, 2005), Golooba-Mutebi and Tollman (2007), and Posel, Kahn, and Walker (2007).
29. Ashforth (2002:128).
30. According to a study conducted in the early 1990s (well before AIDS deaths skyrocketed), healers agreed that when poisoned by isidliso, "the victim becomes thin, loses appetite, coughs continuously as if he/she has tuberculosis, vomits (blood in some cases) and becomes dark in complexion" (G. Oosthuizen, quoted in Ashforth 2002:130).
31. Ashforth (2002:132).
32. Rödlach (2006:111–13).
33. Ashforth (2002:139).
34. Steinberg (2008:131–32).
35. Marwick (1964).
36. More precisely, respondents were asked how much they trusted both health ministers in regard to AIDS with possible response scores ranging from 1 for "not at all" to 5 "very much." The score for trust in Hogan was then subtracted from that for Tshabalala-Msimang. A binary variable was then created, taking a value of 1 for a positive score (indicating that Tshabalala-Msimang was trusted more on AIDS than Hogan) and 0 for scores of zero or below.
37. See Nattrass (2007) and Geffen (2010).
38. The p-value is the probability of the result being randomly generated. Coefficients with three stars indicate that this probability is less than 1%, two stars, less than 5%, and one star, less than 10%. The standard error helps assess the

reliability of the point estimate of the coefficient. We can be 95% sure that the "true" value lies somewhere between the coefficient plus twice the standard error, and the coefficient minus twice the standard error. Thus, in the case of the coefficient on African in Model 1, we can be 95% certain that the true value lies somewhere between 4 and 12.

39. Hofstadter (1965:40).

40. Focus group discussions among survey respondents who did not endorse AIDS conspiracy beliefs suggest that many religiously oriented respondents believe that AIDS is a "punishment from God," and thus it is probably unsurprising that they are less than taken with AIDS origin conspiracy theories than those without such an already handy interpretation. (Focus group discussions were led by Thobani Ncaphayi, Ncdecka Mbune, and Clara Rubincam for the AIDS and Society Research Unit, University of Cape Town.)

41. There are, however, some differences in this regard between black men and women. Regressions run separately on black men and women reveal that black women are 5.5 times as likely, and men 2.5 times as likely, to believe in AIDS conspiracy theories if they also believe that AIDS deaths may be witchcraft-related occult attacks (see Grebe and Nattrass 2011). The link between cultural traditionalism was also stronger for women than men—as was the case in the United States, using a different measure of traditionalism (Klonoff and Landrine 1999:456).

42. Interestingly, there were strong gender differences here. In regressions run separately for black men and women, having heard of the TAC almost triples the odds of endorsing AIDS conspiracies for women, while having no statistically significant effect for men (Grebe and Nattrass 2011). This may be because the TAC's first campaign was of particular relevance to women, i.e., to provide antiretrovirals to help prevent mother-to-child transmission of HIV. Women were thus more likely to come across the TAC (and indeed, most TAC activists are women) and to learn more about and appreciate the power of the science of HIV and develop a critical consciousness toward Mbeki and Tshabalala-Msimang.

43. Farmer (1993:235).

44. Treichler (1999:39).

45. Controlling for other determinants of sexual behavior, belief in AIDS conspiracy theories reduces the odds of using a condom by about a third (Grebe and Nattrass 2011).

46. See Schneider and Fassin (2002) and Fassin (2007).

47. Steinberg (2007).

48. Cohen (1999:70).

49. Ibid., 202.

50. Ibid.
51. Gardell (2002) and Singh (1997).
52. Koech and Obel (1990).
53. Holmberg (2008:153).
54. See "The Angry Politics of Kemron," *Newsweek*, Jan. 4, 1994; available at www .newsweek.com/1993/01/03/the-angry-politics-of-kemron.html.
55. Wittes (1993).
56. Roberts (1992).
57. Whitfield (2000a).
58. Wittes (1993).
59. See "The Angry Politics of Kemron," *Newsweek*, Jan. 4, 1994.
60. Ibid.
61. Wakefield (1997).
62. Dodd (1996). Koech was later suspended from the KEMRI for misappropriation of funds and charged with corruption.
63. Wakefield (1997).
64. See "Farrakhan vows to fight AIDS in Zimbabwe" (by A. Muhammad), posted July 23, 2002; available at www.finalcall.com/peacemission/mlf_aids07-23-2002.htm.
65. Whitfield (2000a).
66. This was known in 1990; see J. James (1990). [["Oral Interferon: Hope or Hype?" In *AIDS Treatment News*, no. 101, Apr. 28; see www.aegis.com/pubs/atn/1990/atn10101.html.]]
67. Correspondence from Martin Delaney, Mar, 5, 2008.

4. SCIENCE, POLITICS, AND CREDIBILITY: DAVID GILBERT FIGHTS AIDS CONSPIRACY BELIEFS IN US PRISONS

1. AIDS deaths in US prisons rose sharply over this period, to peak in 1994 at over 100 AIDS deaths per 100,000 inmates before falling sharply with the advent of new therapies (Spaulding et al. 2002:309). New York state, where Gilbert was incarcerated, had more than double the number of HIV-positive prisoners than any other state (ibid., 306).
2. Correspondence from David Gilbert dated Nov. 26, 2010.
3. See, for example, Bogart and Bird (2003), Bogart and Thorburn (2005), Ross, Essien, and Torres (2006), Bohnert and Latkin (2009), and Bogart, Galvin et al. (2010).
4. See Grebe and Nattrass (2011).
5. Correspondence from David Gilbert dated Nov. 26, 2010.

6. Bratich (2008:9).
7. Fiske (1994:215).
8. Ibid., 191.
9. Bratich (2008:106).
10. Correspondence from David Gilbert dated Nov. 22, 2009.
11. Gilbert (2004b:121–27).
12. See Berger (2006) for a longer and more contextualized version of Gilbert's political history.
13. Correspondence from David Gilbert dated Nov. 26, 2010.
14. Berger (2006:21)
15. See www.kersplebedeb.com/mystuff/profiles/gilbert/aidsconsp.html.
16. Gilbert (2004a). Subsequent page numbers from this work are cited in the text.
17. Bratich (2008:106).
18. Correspondence from David Gilbert dated Nov. 26, 2010.
19. Douglass (1987, 1989).
20. Gilbert (2004a:131–32). Subsequent page numbers from this work are cited in the text.
21. Correspondence from David Gilbert dated Nov. 2, 2009.
22. Bratich (2008:113).
23. Correspondence from David Gilbert dated Nov. 22, 2009.
24. Bratich (2008:117).
25. Bratich presents Graves as if he was a respectable establishment figure, as: "Dr Boyd Graves, Director of AIDS Concerns of the international medical research foundation, Common Cause" (2008:118). This suggests that Bratich had done no investigation into the truly paranoid and fantastical world of Boyd "Ed" Graves—or into the nature and reasons for the failure of his lawsuits (see chapter 2).
26. Barkun (2003:162).
27. See www.healthyworldstore.com/MIRACLE-6-p/miracle-6.htm.
28. For example, in a backnote Bratich writes: "Some health educators are attempting to transform their knee-jerk dismissals of AIDS bio-warfare accounts. . . . Others are devoting websites to debunking these accounts in the name of health (Healthwatcher, http://www.healthwatcher.net/Quackery watch/Horowitz)" (2008:183).
29. Bratich (2008:118).
30. Gilbert (2004a:136).
31. Ibid.
32. Bogart and Thorburn (2005:218).
33. Rubincam (2008:29).
34. Correspondence from David Gilbert dated Nov. 2, 2009.

35. Posted on www.kersplebedeb.com/mystuff/profiles/gilbert/aids_rev.html, undated.
36. Posted on ibid.

5. SCIENCE, CONSPIRACY THEORY, AND THE SOUTH AFRICAN AIDS POLICY TRAGEDY

1. UNAIDS (2010).
2. See, for example, Fourie (2006), Nattrass (2007), Cullinan and Thom (2009), and Geffen (2010).
3. According to Farber (2000), it was a journalist, Anita Allen, who suggested that Mbeki convene a panel and provided suggestions about whom to invite.
4. Moore, quoted in Cherry (2000:405).
5. Garrett (2002).
6. Msomi and Munusamy (2003).
7. For discussions of the Rath case, see Geffen (2010), Thom (2009), Cullinan (2009), and McGregor (2009).
8. For a history of this early period of scientific discovery, see Gallo (2002) and Montagnier (2002).
9. Volberding and Deeks (2010:49).
10. See Ndung'u et al. (2006).
11. Palella et al. (1998), Jordan et al. (2002), Smit et al. (2006); and for reviews of the evidence, see Chigwedere and Essex (2010) and Volberding and Deeks (2010).
12. Broder (2010:10) and Rosen et al. (2010).
13. Farmer et al. (2001).
14. For Haiti, see Farmer et al. (2001), and for South Africa, see WHO (2003), Coetzee et al. (2004), and Steinberg (2008).
15. Connor et al. (1994) and Volmink et al. (2007).
16. Fischl et al. (1987), Fischl et al. (1989), and Richman et al. (1987).
17. See Delaney (2006) for an accessible discussion, and Richman et al. (2009) for more scientific details.
18. Holmberg (2008:161–62).
19. See, for example, Sonnabend (2000) and Schüklenk (2004).
20. Chigwedere et al. (2008:410).
21. Dugger (2008).
22. Papadopulos-Eleopulos et al. (1999).
23. Cherry (2000).
24. "Face to Face with the President," *Sunday Times* (South Africa), Feb. 6, 2000.

25. Papadopulos-Eleopulos (1999). The archive of *Current Medical Research and Opinion* does not provide any links to this supplement; see http://informa healthcare.com/loi/cmo?open=1999#id_1999.
26. Epstein (1996:15).
27. See Cherry (2009) for a discussion of this episode.
28. Paragraphs 120 to 122 of Judge John Sulan's ruling, Supreme Court of South Australia, *R v Parenzee*, Apr. 27, 2007. Available at www.aidstruth.org/documents/ Supreme-Court-of-South-Australia.pdf.
29. Presidential AIDS Advisory Panel Report (PAAPR 2001:14). Subsequent page numbers from this report are cited in the text.
30. Fassin (2007).
31. Wang (2008).
32. See in particular Fassin (2007:129–45).
33. Mbeki (2000b).
34. Fauci (2007).
35. For example, compare Nattrass (2009) and Sawers and Stillwaggon (2010).
36. Nattrass (2009).
37. Fassin (2007:16).
38. See, for example, Latour (2004) and Collins (2009).
39. Collins (2009:31).
40. For the Thai study, see Shaffer et al. (1999), and Brocklehurst (2002) for a review of the early clinical trials.
41. Quoted in the *Citizen*, Feb. 20, 1998, cited in Heywood (2004:107).
42. Nattrass (2004).
43. Mbeki (1999) and Nattrass (2007:54–55).
44. Tshabalala-Msimang, quoted in Heywood (2003:282).
45. This report comes from Rasnick (2000) and cannot be confirmed.
46. WHO (2000).
47. Nattrass (2007).
48. This model is available at www.assa.org.za.
49. Nattrass (2007, 2008a).
50. Chigwedere et al. (2008).
51. Zulu, quoted in Nolan (2007:232).
52. Letter from Zulu quoted in http://oraclesyndicate.twoday.net/stories/3730077. For video footage of Zulu discussing Mbeki's influence, see http://beatit.co .za/beat-it-2000/episode-12.
53. Zulu, quoted in Nolan (2007:233).
54. Nattrass (2007:120–24).
55. Collins and Evans (2002, 2007).
56. See, for example, Latour (1999) and other selected readings in Biagioli (1999).

57. Njabulo Ndebele (2004) and Frank Chikane (see Cullinan 2010) have written strong defenses of Mbeki on the same grounds.

58. Epstein (1996).

59. The early trials prescribed up to 1,500 mg per day when the standard of care today is 500–600 mg per day.

60. As Holmberg points out, the combination of declining effectiveness accompanied by significant side effects resulted in a persistent public perception that AZT was not simply ineffective, but was actually "poison" (2008:157).

61. Palella et al. (1998).

62. Holmberg (2008:171).

63. Brink (1999); see also Brink (2001).

64. Martin (1999).

65. Both biographies of Mbeki indicate that Brink was an important influence on the president (Gumede 2005:158; Gevisser 2007:729), as does Sparks (2003:286).

66. Mbeki (1999).

67. Mbeki (2000a).

68. Collins and Evans (2007); see also Weinel (2010) for a discussion and extension of their approach.

69. "Primary source knowledge" is a level of expertise which Collins and Evans (2007) identify as being above "popular understanding" but below interactional or constitutive expertise. Weinel (2007, 2010) argues that Mbeki may have attained a level of primary source knowledge—but I am not convinced he achieved even that, given his selective reading of the literature.

70. See Weinel (2009).

71. Brink (2009).

72. Campbell (2002:15).

73. Aaronovitch (2009:10–11).

74. "The Durban Declaration," *Nature* 406 (July 6, 2000: 16.

75. Quoted in Van der Vliet (2004:60).

76. Stewart et al. (2000).

77. Delaney et al. (2000).

78. Rybicki et al. (2000).

79. Shenton (2000).

80. The letters between Thabo Mbeki and Tony Leon were tabled in parliament on October 5, 2000.

81. Mankahlana (2000a).

82. Mankahlana (2000b).

83. The quotes in this paragraph come from the "Statement of the National Executive Committee Meeting of the African National Congress," Oct. 3, 2000 (ANC 2000c) and two ANC press releases issued by Smuts Ngonyame, "The

DA Criticism of the TAC's Decision," Oct. 19, 2000 (ANC 2000a) and "HIV and AIDS as an Electioneering Tool," Oct. 23, 2000 (ANC 2000b).

84. Nattrass (2004:66–98).
85. Hensher (2000).
86. Geffen et al. (2003) and Nattrass (2004:99–131).
87. Nattrass and Geffen (2005) and Badri et al. (2006).
88. See, for example, Butler (2005) and Fourie (2006).
89. Nattrass (2008b).
90. Myburgh (2009).
91. Mbcki (1998).
92. This was revealed in court records following a dispute between the Vissers (Myburgh 2009). Mbcki, however, denied that the ANC had a stake in Virodene (Mbeki 1998).
93. Hyden and Lanegran (1993).
94. See Dodd (1996:1688).
95. Jha et al. (2001).
96. Myburgh (2009).
97. In Gevisser (2007:727).
98. Mbeki and Mokaba (2002). The paper was actually anonymous, but as it was circulated by Mokaba and as the electronic version bore Mbeki's electronic signature (see www.health-e.org.za/news/article.php?uid=20031154), it is widely regarded as having been coauthored by Mbeki. Note also that it was Mbeki who sent an updated version to Mark Gevisser.
99. Gevisser (2007:737).
100. Schneider (2002).
101. Sheckels (2004), Lodge (2002), Gevisser (2007).
102. Gevisser (2007:742).
103. Cameron (2005), Mbali (2004), Gevisser (2007), Fassin (2007), Steinberg (2008), and Wang (2008).
104. Mbeki (2001).
105. Mbeki and Mokaba (2002).
106. Wang (2008:4).
107. Marcuse (1955:243).
108. Mbeki and Mokaba (2002:19).
109. Ibid., 47.
110. Mbeki and Mokaba (2002:96).
111. Ibid., 110–11.
112. Fassim and Schneider (2003), Sheckels (2004), Mbali (2004), Fassin (2007), Youde (2007), and Wang (2008).
113. Phillips (2004).
114. Bell (2006).

115. Mtshali (2002).
116. For example, Lieberman (2009:163).
117. Govender (2004, 2009).
118. Kariem, quoted in "ANC Divided Over Dissident AIDS Report," *The Independent* (Mar. 22).
119. See Govender (2009) and Feinstein (2007).
120. Achmat, quoted in Dugger (2008).
121. Gumede (2005:159).
122. Gevisser (2007:735).

6. HERO SCIENTISTS, CULTROPRENEURS, LIVING ICONS, AND PRAISE-SINGERS: AIDS DENIALISM AS COMMUNITY

1. It is worth noting that the "just asking questions" stance is not only common among AIDS denialists, but is characteristic of most conspiracy theorists (Aaronovitch 2009:1).
2. Maggiore (2000:2–3).
3. Presidential AIDS Advisory Panel Report (PAAPR 2001:79, 86).
4. Youde (2007).
5. See Kaplan and Lööw (2002).
6. A placebo, by definition, is treatment that is biomedically ineffective yet nevertheless has a beneficial effect, either because the patient feels more confident and cared for, or because the mind impacts on the body in powerful ways. Collins and Pinch describe it as a "hole in the heart of the science of medicine" and argue that the very fact we have to control for it in clinical trials "shows us how little we know about the body" (Collins and Pinch 2005:18, 33).
7. Hurley (2006), Bausell (2007), and Ernst and Singh (2008).
8. Chan (2008).
9. Thomas, Nicholl, and Coleman (2001), Eisenberg et al. (1997), and Tindle et al. (2005). In the United States, the use of at least one of sixteen listed alternative therapies rose between 1990 and 1997 from 33.8% to 42.1%, with large and significant increases in herbal medicine, massage therapy, the use of megavitamins, folk remedies, and homeopathy. Extrapolating to the general population, total visits to alternative medicine practitioners exceeded visits to primary health care physicians (Eisenberg et al. 1997). This trend did not change between 1997 and 2002 (Tindle et al. 2005).
10. Coward (1989), Paglia (2003), Partridge (2005), and Sedgwick (2004).
11. Astin (1998:1548).
12. Furnham and Forey (1994) and Siahpush (1998).

13. Harding and Stewart (2003:263–64).
14. Aaronovitch (2009:222).
15. James (2000).
16. Stewart et al. (2000).
17. Rethinking AIDS started life as "The Group for the Scientific Reappraisal of the HIV-AIDS Hypothesis," but was restructured in 2006 under the leadership of David Crowe.
18. Kalichman (2009a).
19. This letter from Zulu appears in an article posted by M. Phiri at http://oracle syndicate.twoday.net/stories/3730077/ 15 May 2007.
20. Duesberg, interview with *Spin* magazine (Sept. 1993); see www.duesberg.com/articles/bginterview.html.
21. See, for example, Duesberg (1996), Bialy (2004), and Farber (2006b).
22. See Kalichman (2009a:45–48).
23. Gallo, in interview with Anthony Liversidge, *Spin* magazine (Feb. 1988). Available at www.duesberg.com/articles/index.html.
24. Youde (2007:4).
25. Wainbert said this in an interview; the transcript is available at www.the othersideofaids.com/images/OSATranscript.pdf, p. 20.
26. See also Kalichman (2009a) and Youde (2007).
27. Farber (2006b).
28. See Kalichman (2009a:34–38).
29. Epstein (1996:333).
30. The suspicion originated from a series of newspaper articles by investigative journalist John Crewdson over whether Gallo "stole" the virus from Montagnieur (Cohen 1991). This Watergate-style reporting culminated in a book (Crewdson 2002) which insinuated but never proved the key claim and was subject to a devastating review in *Science* (Delaney 2002).
31. Enquiries into this by the NIH subsequently exonerated Gallo and found that a particularly aggressive French isolate of HIV had contaminated many of the labs, including Montagnieur's and Gallo's, causing confusion (Delaney 2002).
32. Letter to the editor of *Science*, Dec. 1, 2008; see www.rethinkingaids.com/Home/tabid/146/Default.aspx.
33. See the BBC report "Mbeki's Letter to World Leaders," Apr. 20, 2000; available at http://news.bbc.co.uk/1/hi/world/africa/720448.stm.
34. See Geffen (2010) for a discussion of the Khayelitsha trials, the resulting deaths, and the TAC's successful legal battle against Rath.
35. Bialy (2004:180–81).
36. Mullis (1998).

37. Interview posted on Mullis's website; see www.karymullis.com/pdf/kmullis-interview.pdf.

38. See www.theperthgroup.com.

39. See, for example, www.virusmyth.net/aids/award.htm. There you will find arguments by Peter Duesberg that HIV exists, and long, incomprehensible replies by the Perth Group as to why it does not.

40. Author interview with John Moore, Nov. 29, 2010. Moore reports that David Steele, an AIDS denialist lawyer who also used to run an AIDS denialist blog under the pseudonym "Hank Barnes," has been involved in several unsuccessful such cases in the United States. The retired traffic officer Clark Baker (see n. 102) also appears to be involved in legal action entailing AIDS denialist claims.

41. Those who combat AIDS denialism do not generally support criminalizing HIV exposure or transmission, but will contest denialist claims in court regardless of the case.

42. Turner (2006).

43. Gallo (2007).

44. See chapter 5 (at note 28) for the judge's comments on Papadopulos-Eleopulos.

45. Ruling by Judge John Sulan, paragraph 205–6; see www.aidstruth.org/documents/Supreme-Court-of-South-Australia.pdf.

46. These rather tiresome allegations and counter-allegations can be found at www.tig.org.za/TIG_Position_Statement_on_%27HIV%27.htm and www.tig.org.za/RA&RAConference&PGSep1609.pdf, as well as at www.tig.org.za/RA.htm. See also Farber's defense of Rethinking AIDS at http://forum.the truthbarrier.com/2010/02/07/does-parenzees-defense-team-agree-with-the-anti-ra-brigade-about-parenzee-trial-blame/. For commentary by Snout, see http://snoutworld.blogspot.com/2009/11/seriously-dysfunctional-family-of_26.html.

47. Presumably an "excerpt" was selected in order not to alert members of Congress to Mullis's more eccentric claims (such as his alleged experiences with extraterrestrials, glowing raccoons, and other products of his openly admitted use of hallucinatory drugs).

48. Farber (1999).

49. See www.theothersideofaids.com/producer_biographies.html.

50. Smith and Novella (2007:1313).

51. See also www.dr-rath-foundation.org.za/open_letters/open_letter_2005_05_06.htm.

52. See www4.dr-rath-foundation.org/THE_FOUNDATION/the_truth_about_arvs/index.html.

53. See www.gnhealthyliving.com and www.garynull.com/home/category/aids, where Gary Null promotes his videos and alternative health products. His radio shows are available at www.progressiveradionetwork.com/the-gary-null-show-wnye/. For his recent "investigative report on HIV and AIDS," see: http://justiceandunity.org/Gary-Null/GaryNullShow060410Part1.mp3.

54. Hurley (2006:216).

55. See www.garynull.com/home/aids-is-not-a-death-sentence.html.

56. The TAC had a long-running battle against Rath. For the court documents, see www.tac.org.za/community/rath.

57. In 2006, ACT-UP New York wrote to WBAI to request that they not put Gary Null's health show on the air (see www.actupny.org/reports/denialist_gary_null.html), and in 2010 a broader alliance of AIDS activists did the same when the broadcasting station reconsidered the issue again (see www.aids truth.org/news/2010/wbai-do-not-put-gary-nulls-dangerous-show-air-sign). They were, however, unsuccessful.

58. Available at www.duesberg.com/media/gndeath.html.

59. Duesberg, quoted in "The World's Most Reviled Genius," in *Newsweek*, Oct. 9, 2009. Available at www.newsweek.com/id/217015.

60. Campbell (2002:14).

61. See www.healaids.com/.

62. See www.ellner.info/.

63. See www.theothersideofaids.com/images/OSATranscript.pdf, p. 2.

64. See www.robertogiraldo.com/eng/upcoming_events.html.

65. See www.vivoysano.org.mx/. See also www.jornada.unam.mx/2007/02/01/ls-negacionistas.html.

66. Nattrass and Bergman (2007).

67. See http://youtube.com/watch?v=DbFGJwC8xX4 and http://youtube.com/watch?v=TTHhTpmmz_I.

68. See www.theothersideofaids.com/images/OSATranscript.pdf.

69. A photograph of Maggiore and Mbeki was posted at www.neue-medizin.com/maggmbek.jpg .

70. Maggiore (2000).

71. Ibid., 2.

72. Kleinman et al. (1998).

73. Maggiore (2000:1).

74. A fuller discussion of the test results in *House of Numbers* was posted by Jeanne Bergman at www.houseofnumbers.org/Maggiore_s_Labs.html.

75. Maggiore (2000:32). For evidence on the efficacy of antiretroviral treatment, see chapter 5.

76. Ibid., 29–30.
77. Ibid., 30.
78. Farber (2006a).
79. This cover is reproduced at www.sciencebasedmedicine.org/?p=328. The magazine refused me permission to reproduce the cover because "Christine's family does not give permission to use the image in any way that might denigrate her" (per e-mail dated Nov. 10, 2010).
80. Coroner's report no. 2005–03767 for "Scovill, Eliza" available at www.aids truth.org/documents/ejs-coroner-report.pdf.
81. Ornstein and Costello (2005).
82. See www.thebody.com/content/treat/art6573.html.
83. See www.toxi-health.com/consult.html.
84. Bennett (2006).
85. See http://mothering.com/news-bulletins-november-2005.
86. See http://abcnews.go.com/Primetime/print?id=1386737.
87. Farber (2006a).
88. Ibid.
89. Ibid.
90. Wainberg, quoted in Law (2009).
91. Moore and Nattrass (2006).
92. This was posted on the Rethinking AIDS website without my permission; see www.rethinkingaids.com/challenges/moore-maggiore-scovill.html.
93. For a discussion of the scientific evidence, see pp. 180–82 and the URL in preceding note.
94. Most people progress from HIV infection to AIDS within ten years, but 5–15% are able to fight off infection for much longer—a feat scientists believe is genetic (Deeks and Walker 2007; Owen et al. 2010).
95. The participation of others was revealed when some of the advice they were giving her was accidentally copied to me.
96. See interview with Seth Kalichman by B. Goldman, in *The Body* (June 2009). Available at www.thebody.com/content/art52090.html.
97. Maggiore, quoted in Ornstein and Costello (2005). The Los Angeles District Attorney's Office considered charging Maggiore over the death of Eliza Jane but decided against it on the grounds that she had sought medical advice— hence action was taken against the child's doctor instead.
98. This appears on her death certificate; see www.aidstruth.org/new/sites/default/files/maggiore-death-certificate.pdf.
99. Bergman (2010).
100. The source for the original quote is http://deanesmay.com/2008/12/30/what-killed-christine-maggiore/. Elizabeth Ely from Rethinking AIDS also

claimed in a blog post that Maggiore died from the "relentless onslaught" of critical media coverage; see http://mcgilldaily.com/articles/22781.

101. This is discussed at http://denyingaids.blogspot.com/2009/12/hiv-aids-and-one-year-later-no-rest-for.html.

102. Baker runs a right-wing, pro-AIDS denialist blog; see http://exlibhollywood .blogspot.com/. See also www.aidstruth.org/features/2009/clark-baker-ex-cop-and-homophobic-right-wing-blogger.

103. This quotation from Baker may be found at http://mcgilldaily.com/articles/ 22781.

104. See www.aliveandwell.org/html/top_bar_pages/aboutus.html (last accessed Feb. 16, 2011).

105. See www.aidstruth.org/denialism/dead_denialists.

106. For example, David Gorski, an oncologist who publishes one such pro-science website (www.sciencebasedmedicine.org), wrote a detailed discussion and critique of the claims by AIDS denialists about the death of Maggiore and her daughter (www.sciencebasedmedicine.org/?p=328). Seth Kalichman also posted information about her on his blog (http://denyingaids.blogspot .com/2010/07/how-aids-denialism-can-kill-you-part.html) as did the anti-AIDS denialist website www.aidstruth.org (see www.aidstruth.org/news/ 2009/christine-maggiore-died-aids).

107. See http://wearelivingproof.org/.

108. See http://wearelivingproof.org/karri.html and www.aidstruth.org/denialism/ denialists/dead denialists.

109. Posted by Seth Kalichman; see http://denyingaids.blogspot.com/2010/07/ how-aids-denialism-can-kill-you-part.html.

110. Epstein (1996:105–178).

111. These include Celia Farber, John Lauritsen, Anthony Liversidge, Tom Bethel, Gary Null, Elinor Burkett, Neville Hodgkinson, and Joan Shenton; see links to their writings at Duesberg's website (www.duesberg.com/media/index .html).

112. See http://wearelivingproof.org/.

113. Her articles spelling out his views, portraying him sympathetically, raising doubts about AZT, and claiming that there is very little evidence for an African AIDS epidemic, etc., are listed on her wiki page (www.reviewingaids .com/awiki/index.php/Celia_Farber).

114. Farber (2006b).

115. Gallo et al. (2006).

116. This was the "whistleblower award" made under the auspices of the Semmelweis Society, the leadership of which, at the time, had been taken over by AIDS denialists, notably Clark Baker. The award was protested by other

members of the society and related governance issues remain subject to litigation.

117. For an account of the actions taken by activists, see "Denied" (May 16, 2008). Available at www.thebody.com/content/art46788.html?comments=on #commentTop.

118. For example, in an interview for the online zine BookSlut, she read from an article published in the *Lancet* and claimed that it showed that antiretrovirals do not extend the lives of people with AIDS (see www.bookslut.com/features/2006_09_009885.php). The study (May et al. 2006), however, showed nothing of the kind, finding that antiretrovirals had become no more or less effective at reducing AIDS mortality over time. When challenged by bloggers about this blatant misrepresentation of the article, she declined to reply (see www.spectator.co.uk/coffeehouse/5461313/questioning-the-aids-consensus .html).

119. Interview with Celia Farber by Kruglinski (2006).

120. See http://forum.thetruthbarrier.com/2010/04/07/a-reply-to-the-charge-that-aids-denialism-kills-for-aziz-via-truth-barrier-as-link/.

121. Caspe, quoted in Scott and Kaufman (2005).

122. Dwoskin (2009).

123. See www.altheal.org/toxicity/house.htm.

124. Sharav's son died from a fatal reaction to an antipsychotic drug—a personal tragedy which sparked her subsequent actions as a campaigner against any form of waived consent in clinical trials (Schmidt 2008).

125. Quoted in Scott and Kaufman (2005).

126. Ibid.

127. Dwoskin (2009).

128. John Moore forwarded the press release to a senior science journalist, who showed it to the Deputy Director General of the BBC, who then took the complaint forward (author interview with John Moore, November 30, 2010). He also posted the relevant press release and e-mail, as a challenge to the Rethinking AIDS group, at http://scienceblogs.com/aetiology/2007/10/bbc_apologizes_for_promotion_0.php#comment-615391.

129. See http://news.bbc.co.uk/2/hi/programmes/this_world/4038375.stm.

130. See www.vera.org/content/experiences-new-york-city-foster-children-hivaids-clinical-trials.

131. Reported in Dwoskin (2009).

132. See www.houseofnumbers.org/RealAnswersHON.html, and http://www .aidstruth.org/features/2009/real-answers-fake-questions-%E2%80%9Chouse-numbers%E2%80%9D.

133. See www.badscience.net/2009/09/house-of-numbers/.

134. According to the "motion on funding" (see www.tig.org.za/Minutes_RA2006 .htm), "Bob Leppo moved that RA board authorize the RA foundation to make grants for a wider range of purposes, including films and video. Seconded by Charles Geshekter. Funding for each project would still have to be approved by a 2/3 majority of the board. Board members involved in a project would recuse themselves from such decisions. Unanimous agreement. Roberto Giraldo moved that the RA foundation make grants for Brent Leung's film based on available funds. Seconded by Christine Maggiore. Unanimous agreement."

135. These are available at www.houseofnumbers.org/What_Interviewees_Say .html.

136. See www.spectator.co.uk/coffeehouse/5461313/questioning-the-aids-consensus .thtml.

137. Melville (2009).

138. See www.badscience.net/2009/09/house-of-numbers/.

139. Melville (2009).

140. See http://aidsmyth.blogspot.com/.

141. J. T. de Shong runs a website, "dissidents4Dumbees" (see http://dissidents4 dumbees.blogspot.com).

142. See www.blogger.com/profile/00315836146914661895.

143. All these comments are posted at http://blog.newhumanist.org.uk/2009/09/ was-i-conned-by-aids-denialists.html.

144. Melville published this comment in a post linked to an article he subsequently asked Kalichman to write on "How to Spot an AIDS Denialist" (Kalichman 2009b).

145. Kalichman (2009a:xiii–xiv).

7. DEFENDING THE IMPRIMATUR OF SCIENCE: DUESBERG AND THE *MEDICAL HYPOTHESES* SAGA

1. Merton (1957).

2. See, for example, articles in Biagioli (1999).

3. See Collins (1998).

4. Gieryn (1983:781).

5. Ibid. See Nattrass (2011) for a more detailed discussion of boundary work and the related sociology of science.

6. Weinel (2008) argues that there are four criteria to distinguish a counterfeit from a genuine scientific controversy—when one side lacks: conceptual continuity with science; relevant expertise; constitutive research in the area;

and creditable acceptance by the scientific community. While Duesberg does have some relevant expertise, his lack of research in the field of HIV and his rejection by the scientific community for disregarding key evidence places the "controversy" he keeps alive firmly in the area of a counterfeit controversy.

7. Zuckerman and Merton (1971).

8. Ziman (1966:148).

9. Burnham (1990) and Weller (2001).

10. See, for example, Trafimow and Rice (2009); see also *The Scientist* (Aug. 2010:31–35), in which five important papers are discussed which did not make it into top journals because they were rejected by peer reviewers ("Breakthroughs from the Second Tier" by *The Scientist* staff).

11. Suls and Martin 2009: 42.

12. Zuckerman and Merton (1971:96–98).

13. Suls and Martin (2009:46–48) and Akst (2010).

14. Suls and Martin (2009:47).

15. Horobin (1975). See also Charlton (2010) and Cartwright (2010b).

16. Horobin (1975:1).

17. Ibid., 2.

18. This is available at www.rethinkingaids.com/Challenges/Crowe-Scalise-et-al .html.

19. See physics.smu.edu/~pseduo/Intro.

20. See, for example, www.badscience.net/2008/10/more-crap-journals/.

21. Chigwedere et al. (2008).

22. Nattrass (2008a). See also chapter 5, this volume.

23. Geffen (2009) and Cartwright (2010b).

24. Duesberg et al. (2009).

25. Chigwedere and Essex (2010).

26. Crowe, D. (2010).

27. See, for example, Blattner, Gallo, and Temin (1988), Weiss and Jaffe (1990), Gallo (1991), Cohen (1994), O'Brien and Goedert (1996), Moore (1996), Galea and Chermann (1998), Gallo et al. (2006), and Chigwedere and Essex (2010).

28. For example, Duesberg (1996), Duesberg and Rasnick (1998), Duesberg, Koehnlein, and Rasnick (2003), and Duesberg et al. (2009).

29. Winkelstein, in Hughes (1994:131).

30. Moore (1996:722).

31. Duesberg (2007).

32. Donegan et al. (1990).

33. See Cohen (1994).

34. Maddox (1993).

35. Ibid., 109.

36. Chigwedere et al. (2008).
37. Duesberg also wrote to the editor, William Blattner, accusing one of the authors (Max Essex) of having an undisclosed financial interest in a biomedical company and thus supposedly standing to benefit from their defense of the science of antiretrovirals. The complaint was forwarded to Harvard (where Essex is employed) and found to be groundless.
38. In Cartwright (2010a).
39. May et al. (2006).
40. Duesberg et al. (2009:5).
41. Charlton (2010).
42. Ibid.
43. Chigwedere et al. (2008) and Nattrass (2008a).
44. "The Cost of Silence?" *Nature* 456 (Dec. 4): 545.
45. Karim, Coovadia, and Makgoba (2008).
46. Chigwedere and Essex (2010).
47. This letter and list of signatories is available at www.aidstruth.org/sites/aids truth.org/files/NLMLetter-2009.08.05.pdf .
48. See www.badscience.net/2009/09/medical-hypotheses-fails-the-aids-test/.
49. See www.ncbi.nlm.nih.gov/pubmed/19619953 .
50. Charlton, quoted in Cressey (2010).
51. Charlton (2010).
52. See www.badscience.net/2009/09/medical-hypotheses-fails-the-aids-test/.
53. May et al. (2006).
54. See www.badscience.net/2009/09/medical-hypotheses-fails-the-aids-test/.
55. After Charlton was fired as editor, a one-time student of Horobin's and long-standing member of the *Medical Hypotheses* board, Mehar Manku, was appointed editor. He announced that he would "retain the ethos, heritage and unique characteristics of the journal as they were proposed at inception," but that he would be engaging "a medically-qualified Editorial Board" whose members will "look at the premise, originality and plausibility of the hypotheses submitted whilst also ensuring their scientific merit" (Manku 2010:275).
56. Mroz (2010).
57. See, for example, Smith and Novella (2007).

8. THE CONSPIRATORIAL MOVE AND THE STRUGGLE FOR EVIDENCE-BASED MEDICINE

1. Wakefield et al. (1998).
2. Offit (2008:21).

3. Ibid.
4. Boseley (2010). Subsequent reports suggest that some of Wakefield's data was misreported to the point of being fraudulent (Deer 2011).
5. Fraser (2001b).
6. Offit (2008:31–34).
7. Fraser (2001a).
8. For a biting review of the film, see Aaronovitch (2003).
9. Picardie (2002).
10. Offit (2008:184).
11. Fraser (2001b, 2001a).
12. Hargreaves, Lewis, and Speers (2003:42).
13. Cohen 2002.
14. Honan (2003).
15. "Cherie Health Guru Who Believes MMR Jab Is Unnecessary," *Daily Mail* (London), Dec. 26, 2001.
16. Hargreaves, Lewis, and Speers (2003:41–42, emphasis in the original).
17. Ibid., 44.
18. Offit (2008:24).
19. See www.guardian.co.uk/science/2010/jan/28/andrew-wakefield-downfall.
20. Horton, quoted in Offit (2008:58).
21. Ibid.
22. Miller (2010).
23. Harris (2010).
24. Brian Deer's research on the topic is available at http://briandeer.com/wakefield-deer.htm.
25. Institute of Medicine (IOM 2004).
26. Offit (2008:42–44).
27. Ibid., xvii–xviii.
28. See www.generationrescue.org/about/jenny. McCarthy argues that her son was cured through a gluten-free, casein-free diet, vitamin supplementation, and various detoxification strategies followed by behavioral therapy—and notes that medical professionals now say that her son was probably misdiagnosed in the first place, something she does not believe (see J. McCarthy and J. Carrey, "My Son's Recovery from Autism" [2008], atwww.cnn.com/2008/US/04/02/mccarthy.autsimtreatment/index.html).
29. Cited in Greenveld (2010).
30. See J. McCarthy and J. Carrey, "Andrew Wakefield, Scientific Censorship and Fourteen Monkeys" (Feb. 20100 at www.momlogic.com/2010/02/a_statement_from_jenny_mccarth.php.
31. Wakefield et al. (2009).

32. See www.thoughtfulhouse.org/clinical-treatment.php.

33. Angell (2005), Goozner (2004), and Goldacre (2008).

34. See Smith (2005) and Goldacre (2008).

35. Specter (2010).

36. Jüni et al. (2005).

37. Horton (2004).

38. See, for example, Angell (2005) and Goldacre (2008).

39. Cohen (2006).

40. Goldacre (2008:184).

41. Kurtz (2009).

42. Goldacre (2008), Offit (2008), and Kalichman (2009a).

43. Hurley (2006), Ernst and Singh (2008), and Specter (2010).

44. Goldacre was sued by Mattias Rath, the multinational cultropreneur who runs the Rath Health Foundation and claims that his expensive vitamins cure many illnesses including AIDS, bird flu, and cancer. Rath is notorious for conducting illegal "trials" in Khayelitsha in which AIDS patients were encouraged to go off antiretrovirals and onto his high-dose vitamin regimen instead (chapters 5 and 6). Fortunately, Goldacre could rely on the *Guardian* to cover the costs of the trial, which was finally resolved in his favor. Singh, however, was sued in his individual capacity by the British Chiropractic Association for saying that they happily promoted "bogus" therapies. He had to rely on public support for his cause, but fortunately, like Goldacre, ultimately proved successful.

45. These include the group of physicians who participate in a website called "Science-Based Medicine" because they have become "alarmed at the manner in which unscientific and pseudoscientific health care ideas have increasingly infiltrated academic medicine and medicine at large" (www.sciencebased medicine.org), academics like Tara Smith (an epidemiologist), who runs the blog "Aetiology" (http://scienceblogs.com/aetiology), and David Colquhoun (pharmacologist), who publishes "Improbable Science" (www.dcscience.net). Other active and informed bloggers with a scientific background include "Orac," who runs "Respectful Insolence" (http://scienceblogs.com/insolence), and "Gimpy" (http://gimpyblog.wordpress.com). Other sites are dedicated purely to warning people about quackery (notably, www.quackometer.net and www.quackwatch.org).

46. The posse can be found listed at www.badscience.net/index.php?s=posse.

47. See www.badscience.net/2009/07/we-are-more-possible-than-you-can-power fully-imagine/#more-1272.

48. Gieryn (1983).

49. Thompson (2008:135).

50. Ibid., 138–39.
51. Goldacre (2008:207–208).
52. Nyhan and Reifler (2010).
53. Ibid., 307.
54. Manjoo (2008:107).
55. Ibid., 2.
56. Dean (1998:8).
57. Ibid., 9.
58. Barkun (2003:185–87).
59. Campbell (2002:18).
60. Nyhan and Reifler (2010:308).
61. Nyhan and Reifler found that, whereas in 2005 those who supported George W. Bush were more likely to believe that Iraq had weapons of mass destruction after being presented with evidence that it did not (the "backfire" effect of corrective information), in 2006 this effect had disappeared. They suggest that this had to do with broader public acceptance of the fact that Iraq did not have weapons of mass destruction (2010:311–317).

REFERENCES

Aaronovitch, D[avid]. 2003. "A Travesty of Truth." *The Observer*, Dec. 15.

———. 2009. *Voodoo Histories: The Role of the Conspiracy Theory in Shaping Modern History*. New York: River Head Books.

Abalakina-Paap, M. and W. Stephan. 1999. "Beliefs in Conspiracies." *Political Psychology* 20.3: 637–47.

African National Congress (ANC). 2000a. Press Release, "The DA Criticism of the TAC's Decision" (Oct. 19).

———. 2000b. Press Release, "HIV and AIDS as an Electioneering Tool" (Oct. 23).

———. 2000c. "Statement of the National Executive Committee Meeting of the African National Congress" (Oct. 3).

Akst, J. 2010. "I Hate Your Paper." *The Scientist* (Aug.): 36–41.

Andrew, Christopher and Oleg Gordievsky. 1990. *KGB: The Inside Story of Its Foreign Operations from Lenin to Gorbachev*. New York: HarperCollins.

Angell, Marcia. 2005. The Truth about Drug Companies: How They Deceive Us and What to Do about It. New York: Random House.

"The Angry Politics of Kemron," *Newsweek*, Jan. 4, 1994. Available at www.newsweek.com/1993/01/03/the-angry-politics-of-kemron.html.

Appadurai, Arjun. 1996. *Modernity at Large: Cultural Dimensions of Globalization*. Minneapolis: U of Minnesota P.

Ashforth, A[dam]. 2002. "An Epidemic of Witchcraft? The Implications of AIDS for the Post-Apartheid State." *African Studies* 61.2: 121–43.

——. 2005. *Witchcraft, Violence, and Democracy in South Africa*. Chicago: U of Chicago P.

Astin, J. 1998. "Why Patients Use Alternative Medicine: Results of a National Study." *Journal of the American Medical Association* 279.19: 1548–53.

Badri, Motasim, Gary Maartens, Sundhiya Madalia, Linda-Gail Bekker, John Penrod, Robert Platt, Robin Wood, and Eduard Beck. 2006. "Cost-Effectiveness of Highly Active Antiretroviral Therapy in South Africa." *PLoS Medicine* 3.1: 0048–0056.

Barkun, Michael. 2003. *A Culture of Conspiracy: Apocalyptic Visions in Contemporary America*. Berkeley: U of California P.

Barrell, H. 2000. "Mbeki Fingers CIA in AIDS Conspiracy." *Mail and Guardian* (Johannesburg), Oct. 6.

Basham, L. 2003. "Malevolent Global Conspiracy." *Journal of Social Philosophy* 34.1: 91–103.

Bausell, Barker R. 2007. *Snake Oil Science: The Truth about Complementary and Alternative Medicine*. Oxford: Oxford UP.

Bell, T. 2006. "Rath and Company Is an Assault on the Working Class." *Business Report*, Mar. 17.

Bennett, N. 2006. "A Report on Eliza-Jane Scovill's Death, in rebuttal to that of Mohammed Al-Bayati." Version 2.0; see www.aidstruth.org/documents/A_report_on_Eliza_Ver2.pdf.

Berger, Dan. 2006. *Outlaws of America: The Weather Underground and the Politics of Solidarity*. Oakland: AK Press.

Berger, Marléne and Chandré Gould. 2002. *Secrets and Lies: Wouter Basson and South Africa's Chemical and Biological Warfare Programme*. Cape Town: Zebra Press.

Bergman, J. 2010. "The Cult of HIV Denialism." *Achieve Spring*. Available at www.thebody.com/content/art57918.html.

Bertlet, C. 2009. *Toxic to Democracy: Conspiracy Theories, Demonization, and Scapegoating*. Somerville, MA: Political Research Associates.

Biagioli, Mario, ed. 1999. *The Science Studies Reader*. London: Routledge.

Bialy, Harvey. 2004. *Oncogenes, Aneuploidy: A Scientific Life and Times of Peter H. Duesberg*. Berkeley: North Atlantic Books.

Blackstock, Nelson. 1976. *COINTELPRO: The FBI's Secret War on Political Freedom*. New York: Random House.

Blattner, W., R. Gallo, and H. Temin. 1988. "HIV Causes AIDS." *Science* 241: 515–16.

Bogart, L., F. Galvan, G. Wagner, and D. Klein. 2010. "Longitudinal Association of HIV Conspiracy Beliefs with Sexual Risk among Black Males Living with HIV." *AIDS and Behavior*. Published online (DOI: 10.1007/s10461–010–9796–7); see www.springerlink.com/content/1q7622555j53k4j2/.

Bogart, L., S. Kalichman, and L. Simbayi. 2010. Endorsement of genocidal HIV conspiracy as a barrier to HIV testing in South Africa. Unpublished manuscript.

Bogart, L. M. and S. Thorburn. 2005. "Are HIV/AIDS Conspiracy Beliefs a Barrier to HIV Prevention among African Americans?" *Journal of Acquired Immune Deficiency Syndromes* 38. 2: 213–18.

——. 2006. "Relationship of African Americans' Sociodemographic Characteristics to Belief in Conspiracies about HIV/AIDS and Birth Control." *Journal of the National Medical Association* 98.7: 1144–50.

Bogart, L. M. and S. Thorburn Bird. 2003. "Exploring the Relationship of Conspiracy Beliefs about HIV/AIDS to Sexual Behaviors and Attitudes among African-American Adults." *Journal of the National Medical Association* 95.11: 1057–65.

Bogart, L., G. Wagner, F. Galvan, and D. Banks. 2010. Conspiracy beliefs about HIV are related to antiretroviral treatment nonadherence among African American men with HIV. *Journal of Acquired Immune Deficiency Syndromes* 53.5: 648–55.

Bohnert, A. S. and C. A. Latkin. 2009. "HIV Testing and Conspiracy Beliefs Regarding the Origins of HIV among African Americans." *AIDS Patient Care and STDs* 23.9: 759–63.

Boseley, S. 2010. "Andrew Wakefield Found 'irresponsible' by GMC over MMR Vaccine Scare." *The Guardian*, Jan. 29.

Brandon, D., L. Isaac, and T. LaVeist. 2005. "The Legacy of Tuskegee and Trust in Medical care: Is Tuskegee Responsible for Race Differences in Mistrust of Medical Care?" *Journal of the National Medical Association* 97.7: 951–56.

Bratich, Jack. 2008. *Conspiracy Panics: Political Rationality and Popular Culture*. Albany: SUNY Press.

Briggs, C. 2004. "Theorizing Modernity Conspiratorally: Science, Scale, and the Political Economy of Public Discourse in Explanations of a Cholera Epidemic." *American Ethnologist* 31.2: 164–87.

Brink, A[nthony]. 1999. "AZT: A Medicine from Hell." *The Citizen*, Mar. 17.

——. 2001. *Debating AZT: Mbeki and the AIDS Drug Controversy*. Self-published book, available online at www.whale.to/a/brink_b.html.

——. 2009. "Martin Weinel's Critique of Mbeki—Anthony Brink Replies." Mar. 27. Available at www.politicsweb.co.za/politicsweb/view/politicsweb/en/page71619?oid=123061&sn=Detail.

Brocklehurst, P. 2002. "Interventions for Reducing the Risk of Mother to Child Transmission of HIV Infection." *Cochrane Database of Systematic Reviews* 1. Art. No.: CD000102. Published online (DOI: 10.1002/14651858.CD000102).

Broder, S. 2010. "The Development of Antiretroviral Therapy and Its Impact on the HIV-1/AIDS Pandemic." *Antiviral Research* 85: 1–18.

Burnham, J. 1990. "The Evolution of Editorial Peer Review." *Journal of the American Medical Association* 263: 1323–29.

Butler, A. 2005. "South Africa's AIDS Policy: 1994–2004: How Can It Be Explained?" *African Affairs* 104.417: 591–614.

Butt, L. 2005. "'Lipstick Girls' and 'Fallen Women': AIDS and Conspiratorial Thinking in Papua, Indonesia." *Cultural Anthropology* 20.3: 412–42.

Cameron, Edwin. 2005. *A Witness to AIDS.* Cape Town: David Philip.

Campbell, Colin. 2002. "The Cult, the Cultic Milieu, and Secularization." In Kaplan and Lööw, eds., *The Cultic Milieu,* 12–25.

Campsmith, M., P. Rhodes, H. Hall, and T. Green. 2008. "CDC. 2008. HIV Prevalence Estimates—United States." *Mortality and Morbidity Weekly Report* 57.39: 1073–76.

Cantwell, Alan. 1988. *AIDS and the Doctors of Death: An Inquiry into the Origins of the Epidemic.* New York: Aries Rising Press.

——. 1993. *Queer Blood.* New York: Aries Rising Press.

Cartwright, J. 2010a. "AIDS Contrarian Ignored Warnings of Scientific Misconduct." *Nature,* May 4. Published online (DOI: 10.1038/news.2010.210).

——. 2010b. "Unconventional Thinkers or Recklessly Dangerous Minds?" *Times Higher Education,* May 6; see www.timeshighereducation.co.uk/story.asp?story code=411468.

Chan, E. 2008. "Quality of Efficacy Research in Complementary and Alternative Medicine." *Journal of the American Medical Association* 299.2: 2685–86.

Charlton, B. 2010. "Without Prejudice." *Times Higher Education,* May 6.

Cherry, M. 2000. "South Africa Turns to Research in the Hope of Settling AIDS Policy." *Nature* 405 (May): 105–106.

——. 2009. "The President's Panel." In Cullinan and Thom, eds., *The Virus, Vitamins and Vegetables,* 16–35.

Chigwedere, P. and M. Essex. 2010. "AIDS Denialism and Public Health Practice." *AIDS and Behavior* 14.2: 237–47.

Chigwedere, P., G. Seage, S. Gruskin, T. Lee, and M. Essex. 2008. "Estimating the Lost Benefits of Antiretroviral Drug Use in South Africa." *Journal of Acquired Immune Deficiency Syndromes* 49: 410–15.

Chirimuuta, Richard and Rosalind Chirumuuta. 1989. *AIDS, Africa and Racism.* London: Free Association Books.

Chitnis, A., D. Rawls, and J. Moore. 2000. "Origin of HIV Type 1 in Colonial French Equitorial Africa?" *AIDS Research and Human Retroviruses* 16.1: 5–8.

Chomsky, Noam. 1976. "Introduction." In N. Blackstock, *COINTELPRO: The FBI's Secret War on Political Freedom,* 3–26. New York: Random House.

Clark, A., J. Mayben, C. Hartman, M. Kallen, and T. Giordano. 2008. Conspiracy beliefs about HIV infection are common but not associated with delayed diagnosis or adherence to care. *AIDS Patient Care and STDs* 22.9: 753–59.

Clarke, S. 2002. "Conspiracy Theories and Conspiracy Theorizing." *Philosophy of the Social Sciences* 32: 131–50.

Cochrane, T. 1987. "The Concept of Ecotypes in American Folklore." *Journal of Folklore Research* 24: 33–55.

Coetzee, D., K. Hildebrand, A. Boulle, G. Maartens, F. Louis, V. Labatala, H. Reuter, N. Ntwana, and E. Goemaere. 2004. "Outcomes after Two Years of Providing Antiretroviral Treatment in Khayelitsha, South Africa." *AIDS* 18: 887–95.

Cohen, Cathy. 1999. *The Boundaries of Blackness: AIDS and the Breakdown of Black Politics*. Chicago: U of Chicago P.

Cohen, J. 1991. "Science Journalist as Investigator." *Science* 254: 946–49.

——. 1994. "The Duesberg Phenomenon." *Science* 266: 1642–49.

——. 2000a. "The Hunt for the Origin of AIDS." *Atlantic Monthly* (Oct.).

——. 2000b. "Vaccine Theory of AIDS Origins Disputed at Royal Society." *Science* 2879: 1850–51.

——. 2006. "Pharmanoia: Coming to a Clinical Trial Near You." *Slate* (Feb. 21). Available at www.slate.com/id/2136721/.

Cohen, N. 2002. "Ev'rybody Must Get Stones." *The Observer*, Dec. 8.

Collins, H. 1998. "The Meaning of Data: Open and Closed Evidential Cultures in the Search for Gravitational Waves." *American Journal of Sociology* 104.2: 293–338.

——. 2009. "We Cannot Live by Scepticism Alone." *Nature* 458: 30–31.

Collins, H[arry]. and R[obert]. Evans. 2002. "The Third Wave of Science Studies: Studies of Expertise and Experience." *Social Studies of Science* 32.2: 235–96.

——. 2007. *Expertise: A New Analysis*. Chicago: U of Chicago P.

Collins, Harry and Trevor Pinch. 2005. *Dr. Golem: How to Think about Medicine*. Chicago: U of Chicago P.

Comaroff, Jean and John Comaroff. 1993. "Introduction." In Jean Comaroff and John Comaroff, eds., *Modernity and Its Malcontents: Ritual and Power in Postcolonial Africa*, xi–xxxiii. Chicago: U of Chicago P.

——. 2002. "Alien-Nation: Zombies, Immigrants and Millennial Capitalism." *South Atlantic Quarterly* 101.4: 779–805.

Connor, E., R. Sperling, R. Gelber, P. Kiselev, G. Scott, M. O'Sullivan, R. VanDyke, M. Bey, W. Shearer, R. Jacobson, E. Jimez, E. O'Neill, B. Bazin, J. Delfraissy, M. Culnane, R. Coombs, M. Elkins, J. Moye, P. Stratton, and J. Balsley for the Pediatric AIDS Clinical Trials Group Protocol 076 Study Group. 1994. "Reduction of Maternal-Infant Transmission of Human Immunodeficiency Virus Type 1 with Zidovudine Treatment." *New England Journal of Medicine* 331.18: 1173–80.

Cooper, William. 1991. *Behold a Pale Horse*. Flagstaff, AZ: Light Technology.

"The Cost of Silence." 2008. *Nature* 456 (Dec. 4): 545.

Coward, R. 1989. *The Whole Truth: The Myth of Alternative Medicine*. London: Faber and Faber.

Cressey, D. 2010. "Editor Says No to Peer Review for Controversial Journal." *Nature* (Mar. 18); see www.nature.com/news/2010/100318/full/news.2010.132 .html.

Crewdson, John. 2002. *Science Fictions: A Scientific Mystery, a Massive Cover-up, and the Dark Legacy of Robert Gallo*. New York: Little, Brown.

Crocker, J., R. Luhtanen, S. Broadnax, and B. Blaine. 1999. "Belief in US Government Conspiracies Against Blacks among Black and White College Students: Powerlessness or System Blame?" *Personality and Social Psychology Bulletin* 25: 941–53.

Crowe, D. 2010. "The Potemkin Village of Essex and Chigwedere." Posted on The Truth Barrier (Mar. 19, 2010); see www.thetruthbarrier.com/essays/84-david-crowe/169-the-potemkin-village-of-essex-and-chigwedere.

Cullinan, Kerry. 2009. "Government's Strange Bedfellows." In Cullinan and Thom, eds., *The Virus, Vitamins and Vegetables*, 91–111.

———. 2010. "Frank Chikane's Whitewash of Mbeki Is a Historical Disgrace" (Nov. 8). Available at www.health-e.org.za/news/article.php?uid=20033000.

Cullinan, Kerry and Anso Thom, eds. 2009. *The Virus, Vitamins and Vegetables*. Aukland Park (Johannesburg): Jacana.

Curtis, T. 1992. "The Origin of AIDS." *Rolling Stone* 626: 54–59.

Dalton, H. 1989. "AIDS in Blackface." *Daedalus* 118.3: 205–228.

Darrow, W., J. Montanea, and H. Gladwin. 2009. "AIDS-related Stigma among Black and Hispanic Young Adults." *AIDS and Behavior* 13: 1178–88.

Dean, Jodi. 1998. *Aliens in America: Conspiracy Cultures from Outerspace to Cyberspace*. Ithaca, NY: Cornell UP.

Deeks, S. and B. Walker. 2007. "Human Immunodeficiency Virus Controllers: Mechanisms of Durable Virus Control in the Absence of Antiretroviral Therapy." *Immunity* 27.3: 406–416.

Deer, B. 2011. "How the Case Against the MMR Vaccine Was Fixed." *British Medical Journal* 34: c5347.

Delaney, M. 2002. "Double Jeopardy for Gallo." *Science* 296: 1615–16.

———. 2006. "History of HAART—The True Story of How Effective Multi-drug Therapy Was Developed for Treatment of HIV disease" *Retrovirology* 3 (Supp. 1): S1–S6.

Delaney, M. (et al.). 2000. "Why are AIDS dissidents still making 15-year-old, long-refuted claims?" *Nature* 408 (Nov. 16): 287. The letter was also signed by L. Grinberg, M. Harrington, L. Morris, M. Wainberg, and J. Moore.

DeParle, J. 1990. "Talk of Government Being Out to Get Blacks Falls on More Attentive Ears." *New York Times*, Oct. 29.

Dodd, R. 1996. "Patients Sue the 'AIDS-cure' Kenyan Scientist." *The Lancet* 347: 1688.

Donegan, E., M. Stuart, J. Niland, H. Sacks, A. Stanley, S. Dietrich, C. Faucett, M. Fletcher, S. Kleinman, E. Operskalski, H. Perkins, J. Pindyck, E. Schiff, D. Stites, P. Tomasulo, J. Mosley, and Transfusion Safety Group. 1990. "Infection with Human Immunodeficiency Virus Type 1 (HIV-1 among Recipients of Antibody-Positive Blood Donations." *Annals of Internal Medicine* 113.10: 733–39.

Douglass, William Campbell. 1987. "W.H.O. Murdered Africa (The Man-Made Origin of AIDS)." Widely circulated manuscript. Available at www.conspiracy planet.com/channel.cfm?channelid=34&contentid=2095.

——. 1989. *AIDS: The End of Civilisation.* A & B Distributors.

Duesberg, Peter. 1996. *Inventing the Aids Virus.* Washington, D.C.: Regnery.

——. 2007. "Chromosomal Chaos and Cancer." *Scientific American* 296.5: 52–59.

Duesberg, P., C. Koehnlein, and D. Rasnick. 2003. "The Chemical Bases of the Various AIDS Epidemics: Recreational Drugs, Anti-viral Chemotherapy and Malnutrition." *Journal of Biosciences* 28: 383–412.

Duesberg, P., J. Nicholson, D. Rasnick, C. Fiala, and H. Bauer. 2009. "WITH-DRAWN: HIV-AIDS Hypothesis Out of Touch with South African AIDS— A New Perspective." *Medical Hypotheses*; see www.sciencedirect.com/science/article/pii/S0306987709004472.

Duesberg, P. and D. Rasnick. 1998. "The AIDS Dilemma: Drug Diseases Blamed on a Passenger Virus." *Genetica* 104: 85–132.

Dugger, C. 2008. "Study Cites Toll of AIDS Policy in South Africa." *New York Times*, Nov. 26.

"The Durban Declaration." 2000. *Nature* 406 (July): 15–16.

Dwoskin, E. 2009. "The AIDS-Babies-as-Guinea-Pigs Story Is Finally Over. Right?" *Village Voice*, Apr. 1. Available at www.villagevoice.com/2009-04-01/news/the-aids-babies-as-guinea-pigs-story-is-finally-over-right/.

Eisenberg, D., R. Davis, S. Ettner, S. Appel, S. Wilkey, M. Van Rompay, and R. Kessler. 1997. "Trends in Alternative Medicine Use in the United States, 1990–1997." *Journal of the American Medical Association* 280.18: 1569–75.

Elswood, B. and R. Stricker. 1994. "Polio Vaccines and the Origin of AIDS." *Medical Hypotheses* 42: 347–54.

Epstein, Steven. 1996. *Impure Science: AIDS, Activism, and the Politics of Knowledge.* Berkeley: U of California P.

Ernst, Edzard and Simon Singh. 2008. *Trick or Treatment?* New York: Norton.

Evans-Pritchard, Edward E. 1937. *Witchcraft, Oracles and Magic among the Azande.* Oxford: Clarendon Press.

Farber, C. 1999. "Ignoring the Flames." *Impression* (Aug.). Available at www.virus myth.com/aids/hiv/cfflames.htm.

——. 2000. "AIDS and South Africa: A Contrary Conference in Pretoria." *New York Press*, May 25; see www.virusmyth.net/aids/data/cfmbeki.htm.

——. 2006a. "A Daughter's Death, a Mother's Survival." *LA City Beat*, June 8. Available at www.lacitybeat.com/article/php?id=3887&IssueNum=157.

——. 2006b. "Out of Control: AIDS and the Corruption of Medical Science." *Harper's* (Mar.): 37–52.

Farmer, Paul. 1993. *AIDS and Accusation: Haiti and the Geography of Blame*. Berkeley: U of California P.

Farmer, P. F., J. Léandre, J. Mukherjee, M. Claude, P. Nevil, M. Smith-Fawzi, S. Koenig, A. Castro, M. Becerra, and J. Sachs. 2001. "Community-Based Approaches to HIV Treatment in Resource-Poor Settings." *The Lancet* 358.9279: 404–409.

Fassin, Didier. 2007. *When Bodies Remember: Experiences and Politics of AIDS in South Africa*. Berkeley: U of California P.

Fassin, D. and H. Schneider. 2003. "The Politics of AIDS in South Africa: Beyond the Controversies." *British Medical Journal* 326 (Mar.): 495–97.

Fauci, A., 2007. "Pathogenesis of HIV Disease: Opportunities for New Prevention Interventions." *Clinical Infectious Diseases* 45 (Supp. 4): S206–S212.

Feinstein, Andrew. 2007. *After the Party: A Personal and Political Journey Inside the ANC*. Cape Town: Jonathan Ball.

Fine, G. 1992. "Rumors of Apartheid: The Ecotypification of Contemporary Legends in the New South Africa." *Journal of Folklore Research* 29.1: 53–71.

Finnegan, W. 2001. "The Poison Keeper: Biowarrior, Brilliant Cardiologist, War Criminal, Spy—Can a Landmark Trial in South Africa Reveal Who Wouter Basson Really Was?" *The New Yorker* (Jan. 15): 58.

Fishl, M. et al. 1987. "The Efficacy of Azidothymidine (AZT) in the Treatment of Patients with AIDS and AIDS-related Complex: A Double-blind, Placebo-controlled Trial." *New England Journal of Medicine* 317: 185–281.

Fischl, M. et al. 1989. "Prolonged Zidovudine Therapy in Patients with AIDS and Advanced AIDS-related Complex. AZT Collaborative Working Group." *Journal of the American Medical Association* 262: 2405–2410.

Fiske, John. 1994. *Media Matters: Everyday Culture and Political Change*. Minneapolis: U of Minnesota P.

Fourie, Peter. 2006. *The Political Management of HIV and AIDS in South Africa: One Burden Too Many?* New York: Palgrave Macmillan.

Fraser, L. 2001a. "Parents Left Stunned as MMR Doctor Is Forced Out." *The Telegraph*, Dec. 2.

——. 2001b. "Shame on Officials Who Say MMR Is Safe." *The Telegraph*, Jan. 21.

Frazier, Kendrick, ed. 2009. *Science Under Siege: Defending Science, Exposing Pseudoscience*. New York: Prometheus Books.

Furnham, A. and J. Forey. 1994. "The Attitudes, Behaviours and Beliefs of Patients of Conventional vs Complementary (Alternative) Medicine." *Journal of Clinical Psychology* 50: 458–69.

Galea, P. and J. Chermann. 1998. "HIV as the Cause of Aids and Associated Diseases." *Genetica* 104: 133–42.

Gallo, Robert. 1991. *Virus Hunting: AIDS, Cancer, and the Human Retrovirus—A Story of Scientific Discovery*. New York: Basic Books.

——. 2002. "The Early Years of HIV/AIDS." *Science* 298.5599: 1728–30.

——. 2007. Testimony to the Australian Court of Criminal Appeal in the Andre Parenzee Case, Feb. 12. Available at http://aras.ab.ca/articles/legal/Gallo-Transcript.pdf.

Gallo, R., N. Geffen, G. Gonsalves, R. Jeffries, D. Kuritzkes, B. Mirken, J. Moore, and J. Safrit. 2006. "Errors in Celia Farber's March 2006 article in Harpers Magazine." Posted at www.aidstruth.org/denialism/harpers-farber#a1.

Gallo, R., P. Sarin, P. Allen, W. Newton, E. Priori, J. Bowen, and L. Dmochowski. 1971. "Reverse Transcriptase in Type C Virus Particles of Human Origin." *Nature New Biology* 232: 140–42.

Gamble, V. 1997. "Under the Shadow of Tuskegee: African Americans and Health Care." *American Journal of Public Health* 87.11: 1773–78.

Gardell, Mattias. 2002. "Black and White Unite in Fight?" In Kaplan and Lööw, eds., *The Cultic Milieu*, 152–92.

Garrett, L. 2002. "Anti-HIV Drug Poison, Summit Told." *The Age*, July 9. Available at www.theage.com.au/articles/2002/07/08/1025667115671.html.

Geffen, N[athan]. 2009. "Justice after AIDS Denialism: Should There be Prosecutions and Compensation?" *Journal of Acquired Immune Deficiency Syndromes* 51.4: 454–55.

——. 2010. *Debunking Delusions: The Inside Story of the Treatment Action Campaign*. Cape Town: Jacana Press.

Geffen, N. and E. Cameron. 2009. *The Deadly Hand of Denial: Governance and Politically-instigated AIDS Denialism in South Africa*. Centre for Social Science Research, Working Paper No. 257, University of Cape Town.

Geffen, Nathan, Nicoli Nattrass, and Chris Raubenheimer. 2003. "The Cost of HIV Prevention and Treatment Interventions in South Africa." Centre for Social Science Research, Working Paper No. 28, University of Cape Town.

Geschiere, Peter. 1997. *The Modernity of Witchcraft: Politics and the Occult in Postcolonial Africa*. Charlottesville: UP of Virginia.

Gevisser, Mark. 2007. *Thabo Mbeki: The Dream Deferred*. Johannesburg: Jonathan Ball.

Gieryn, T. 1983. "Boundary-work and the Demarcation of Science from Non-Science: Strains and Interests in Professional Ideologies of Scientists." *American Sociological Review* 48: 781–95.

Gilbert, David. 2004a. "AIDS Conspiracy Theories: Tracking the Real Genocide" (1996). In Gilbert, *No Surrender*, 129–50. Orig. published in 1996 in *Covert Action Quarterly*; see www.kersplebedeb.com/mystuff/profiles/gilbert/aidsconsp.html.

——. 2004b. *No Surrender: Writings from an Anti-Imperialist Political Prisoner.* Montreal: Abraham Guillen Press.

Goertzel, T. 1994. "Belief in Conspiracy Theories." *Political Psychology* 15.4: 731–42.

Goldacre, Ben. 2008. *Bad Science.* London: Fourth Estate.

Goldstuck, Arthur. 1990. *The Rabbit in the Thorn Tree: Modern Myths and Legends of South Africa.* London: Penguin.

Golooba-Mutebi, F. and S. Tollman. 2007. "Confronting HIV/AIDS in a South African Village: The Impact of Health-Seeking Behaviour." *Scandinavian Journal of Public Health* 35 (Supp. 69): 175–80.

Goozner, Merrill. 2004. *The $800 Million Pill: The Truth Behind the Cost of New Drugs.* Berkeley: U of California P.

Govender, P[regs]. 2004. "Experiments in a Politics of Love and Courage, Ruth First Memorial Lecture." *Network News* (July): 9–12. Available at www.getnet .org.za/Network_news_july2004.pdf.

——. 2009. "Love, Courage, Insubordination and HIV/AIDS Denialism." In Cullinan and Thom, *The Virus, Vitamins and Vegetables*, 36–57.

Graves, Boyd E. 2001. *State Origin: The Evidence of the Laboratory Birth of AIDS.* National Organization for the Advancement of Humanity and Zygote Media, Abilene, KS.

Grebe, E. and N. Nattrass. 2011. "AIDS Conspiracy Beliefs and Unsafe Sex in Cape Town." Published online in *AIDS and Behavior* (May 3) (DOI: 10.1007/ s10461-011-9958-2).

Greenveld, K. T. 2010. "The Autism Debate: Who's Afraid of Jenny McCarthy?" *Time*, Feb. 25. Available at www.time.com/time/nation/article/0,8599,1967796,00 .html.

Gumede, William. 2005. *Thabo Mbeki and the Battle for the Soul of the ANC.* Cape Town: Zebra Press.

Gwata F. 2009. "Traditional Male Circumcision: What Is Its Socio-Cultural Significance among Young Xhosa Men?" Centre for Social Science Research, Working Paper No. 264, University of Cape Town.

Harding, S. and K. Stewart. 2003. "Anxieties of Influence: Conspiracy Theory and Therapeutic Culture in Millennial America." In Sanders and West, eds., *Transparency and Conspiracy*, 258–85.

Hargreaves, I., J. Lewis, T. Speers. 2003. "Towards a Better Map: Science, the Public and the Media." Report published by the Economic and Social Research Council. Available at www.esrc.ac.uk/_images/towards_a_better_map_tcm8-13558.pdf.

Harris, G. 2010. "Journal Retracts 1998 Paper Linking Autism to Vaccines." *New York Times*, Feb. 2.

Harris, Robert and Jeremy Paxman. 1982. *A Higher Form of Killing: The Secret Story of Gas and Germ Warfare*. London: Chatto and Windus.

Hatch, R. 2003. "Cancer Warfare." In Ellen Ray and William Schaap, eds., *Bioterror: Manufacturing Wars the American Way*, 18–28. Melbourne and New York: Ocean Press.

Hellinger, D. 2003. "Paranoia, Conspiracy, and Hegemony in American Politics." In Sanders and West, eds., *Transparency and Conspiracy*, 204–232.

Henderson, P. 2005. "A Gift Without Shortcomings: Healers Negotiating the Intersection of the Local and the Global in the Context of AIDS." *Social Dynamics* 31.2: 24–54.

Hensher, Martin. 2000. "Confidential Briefing: The Costs and Cost Effectiveness of Using Nevirapine or AZT for the Prevention of Mother to Child Transmission of HIV—Current Best Estimates for South Africa," Apr. 19 (unpublished).

Herrera, F., R. Adamson, and R. Gallo. 1970. "Uptake of Transfer Ribonucleic Acid by Normal and Leukemic Cells." *Proceedings of the National Academy of Sciences* 67.4: 1943–50.

Heywood, M. 2003. "Preventing Mother to Child HIV Transmission in South Africa: Background, Strategies and Outcomes of the Treatment Action Campaign Case Against the Minister of Health." *South African Journal of Human Rights* 19: 278–315.

——. 2004. "The Price of Denial." *Development Update* 5.3: 93–122.

Hitchens, Christopher. 1993. *For the Sake of Argument*. London: Verso.

Hofstadter, Richard. 1965. "The Paranoid Style in American Politics" (orig. 1952). In Hofstadter, *The Paranoid Style in American Politics and Other Essays*. New York: Knopf.

Holmberg, Scott. 2008. *Scientific Errors and Controversies in the US HIV/AIDS Epidemic: How They Slowed Advances and Were Solved*. Westport, CT: Praeger.

Honan, C. 2003. "Cherie is the most delightful caring person and so is Tony." *The Telegraph*, Mar. 28.

Hooper, Edward. 2000. *The River: A Journey to the Source of HIV and AIDS*. Boston: Back Bay Books.

——. 2003. "Dephlogistication, Imperial Display, Apes, Angels, and the Return of Monsieur Émile Zola: New Developments in the Origins of AIDS Controversy, including some observations about the ways in which the scientific establishment may seek to limit open debate and flow of information on 'difficult' issues." Available at www.uow.edu.au/~/bmartin/dissent/documents/AIDS/Hooper03/Hooper03.pdf.

Horobin, D. 1975. "Ideas in Biomedical Science: Reasons for the Foundation of *Medical Hypotheses*." *Medical Hypotheses* 1.1: 1–2.

Horowitz, Leonard. 1996. *Emerging Viruses: AIDS and Ebola—Nature, Accident, or Intentional?* Standpoint, ID: Tetrahedron.

Horton, R. 2004. "Vioxx, the Implosion of Merck, and Aftershocks at the FDA." *The Lancet* 364.9540: 1995–96.

Hughes, S. 1994. Interview with Warren Winkelstein (Oct. 26). Available at http://content.cdlib.org/view?docId=kt7w10060s&query=&brand=calisphere.

Hurley, Dan. 2006. *Natural Causes: Death, Lies, and Politics in America's Vitamin and Herbal Supplement Industry.* New York: Broadway Books.

Hutchinson, A., E. Begley, P. Sullivan, H. Clark, B. Boyett, and S. Kellerman. 2007. "Conspiracy Beliefs and Trust in Information about HIV/AIDS among Minority Men Who Have Sex with Men." *Journal of Acquired Immune Deficiency Syndromes* 45.5: 603–605.

Hyden, G. and K. Lanegran. 1993. "AIDS, Policy and Politics: East Africa in Comparative Perspective." *Policy Studies Review* 12.1–2 (Spring–Summer): 47–65.

Iliffe, John. 2006. *The African AIDS Epidemic: A History.* Cape Town: James Currey and Double Storey.

Institute of Medicine (IOM). 2004. "Immunization Safety Review: Vaccines and Autism." Available at www.iom.edu/Reports/2004/Immunization-Safety-Review-Vaccines-and-Autism.aspx.

James, J. 1990. "Oral Interferon: Hope or Hype?" In *AIDS Treatment News* 101, Apr. 28; see www.aegis.com/pubs/atn/1990/atn10101.html.

——. 2000. "AIDS Denialists: How to Respond." *AIDS Treatment News* 342. Available at www.aegis.org/pubs/atn/2000/atn34210.html.

Jameson, Fredric. 1991. *Postmodernism; Or, The Cultural Logic of Late Capitalism.* Durham, NC: Duke UP.

Jha, P., L. Vaz, F. Plummer, N. Nagelkerke, B. Willbond, E. Ngugi, S. Moses, G. John, R. Nduati, K. MacDonald, and S. Berkley. 2001. "The Evidence Base for Interventions to Prevent HIV Infection in Low- and Middle-Income Countries." CMH Working Paper No. WG 5:2. Available at www.emro.who.int/cbi/PDF/HIV_Infection.pdf

Johnson, Loch. 1985. *A Season of Inquiry: The Senate Intelligence Investigation.* Lexington: The UP of Kentucky.

Jordan, R., L. Gold, C. Cummins, and C. Hyde. 2002. "Systematic Review and Meta-analysis of Evidence for Increasing Numbers of Drugs in Antiretroviral Combination Therapy." *British Medical Journal* 324: 1–10.

Jüni, P., Linda Nartey, Stephan Reichenbach, Rebekka Sterchi, Paul A. Dieppe, and Matthias Egger. 2004. "Risk of Cardiovascular Events and Rofecoxib: Cumulative Meta-analysis." *The Lancet* 364.9450: 2021–29.

Kalichman, Seth. 2009a. *Denying AIDS: Conspiracy Theories, Pseudoscience, and Human Tragedy.* New York: Springer.

——. 2009b. "How to Spot an AIDS Denialist." *New Humanist* 124.6 (Dec.). Available at http://newhumanist.org.uk/2165/how-to-spot-an-aids-denialist.

Kalichman, S. and L. Simbayi. 2004. "Traditional Beliefs About the Cause of AIDS and AIDS-Related Stigma in South Africa." *AIDS Care* 16.5: 572–80.

Kaplan, Jeffrey and Heléne Lööw, eds. 2002. *The Cultic Milieu: Oppositional Subcultures in an Age of Globalization*. New York: AltaMira Press.

Karim, S., H. Coovadia, and M. Makgoba. 2008. "Scientists Stand by Decision to Join Mbeki's Panel." *Nature* 457: 379.

Katz, R., S. Kegeles, N. Kressin, L. Green, S. James, M. Wang, S. Russell, and C. Claudio. 2008. "Awareness of the Tuskegee Syphilis Study and the US Presidential Apology and Their Influence on Minority Participation in Biomedical Research." *American Journal of Public Health* 98.6: 1137–42.

Kauffman, Kyle and David Lindauer, eds. *AIDS and South Africa: The Social Expression of a Pandemic*. New York: Palgrave Macmillan.

Keeley, B. 1999. "Of Conspiracy Theories." *Journal of Philosophy* 96.3: 109–126.

———. 2003. "Nobody Expects the Spanish Inquisition. More Thoughts on Conspiracy Theory." *Journal of Social Philosophy* 34.1: 104–110.

Kelly, M. 1995. "The Road to Paranoia." *The New Yorker*, June 19: 60–75.

Kessler, R., G. Andrews, L. Colpe, E. Hiripi, D. Mroczek, S. Normand, E. Walters, and A. Zaslavsky. 2002. "Short Screening Scales to Monitor Population Prevalences and Trends in Non-Specific Psychological Distress." *Psychological Medicine* 32: 959–76.

Kincaid, C. 2008. "Jeremiah Wright's Controversial AIDS Charge." *Accuracy in Media* (Apr. 28); see www.aim.org/aim-column/jeremiah-wrights-controversial-aids-charge.

Kirk, P. 2000. "Govt AIDS Nut Linked to Ku Klux Klan." *Mail and Guardian* (Johannesburg), Sept. 8.

Kleinman, S., M. Busch, L. Hall, R. Thomson, S. Glynn, D. Gallahan, H. Ownby, and A. Williams. 1998. "False-Positive HIV-1 Test Results in a Low-risk Screening Setting of Voluntary Blood Donation: Retrovirus Epidemiology Donor Study." *Journal of the American Medical Association* 280.12: 1080–85.

Klonoff, E. and H. Landrine. 1999. "Do Blacks Believe That HIV/AIDS Is a Government Conspiracy Against Them?" *Preventative Medicine* 28: 451–57.

Knight, Peter. 2002. "Introduction: A Nation of Conspiracy Theorists." In Knight, ed., *Conspiracy Nation*, 1–20.

Knight, Peter, ed. *Conspiracy Nation: The Politics of Paranoia in Postwar America*. New York: NYU Press.

Koech, D. and A. Obel. 1990. "Efficacy of Kemron (low dose oral natural human interferon alpha) in the management of HIV-1 infection and acquired immune deficiency syndrome (AIDS)." *East African Medical Journal* 67.7 (Supp. 2): SS64–SS70.

Koehler, John. 1999. *Stasi: The Untold Story of the East German Secret Police*. Boulder: Westview.

Korber, B., M. Muldoon, J. Theiler, R. Gao, A. Lapedes, B. Hahn, S. Wolinsky, and T. Bhattacharya. 2000. "Timing the Ancestor of the HIV-1 Pandemic Strains." *Science* 288.5472: 1789–96.

Kruglinski, S. 2006. "Questioning the HIV Hive Mind" (interview with Celia Farber). *Dicober* (Oct. 19).

Kurtz, P. 2009. "Science and the Public: Summing Up Thirty Years of the *Skeptical Inquirer*." In Frazier, ed., *Science Under Siege*, 19–33.

Kyle, W. 1992. "Simian Retroviruses, Polio-Vaccine and the Origin of AIDS." *The Lancet* 339: 600–601.

Lapidos, J. 2008. "The AIDS Conspiracy Handbook: Jeremiah Wright's Paranoia, in Context." *Slate Explainer* (Mar. 19); see www.slate.com/id/2186860.

Latour, B. 1999. "Give Me a Laboratory and I Will Raise the World." In Biagioli, ed., *The Science Studies Reader*, 258–75.

——. 2004. "Why Has Critique Run Out of Steam? From Matters of Fact to Matters of Concern." *Critical Inquiry* 30 (Winter): 225–48.

Law, S. 2009. "In Denial." *McGill Daily* (Montreal), Nov. 16; see http://mcgilldaily .com/articles/22781.

Lieberman, Evan. 2009. *Boundaries of Contagion: How Ethnic Politics Have Shaped Government Responses to AIDS*. Princeton: Princeton UP.

Lodge, Tom. 2002. *Politics in South Africa: From Mandela to Mbeki*. Bloomington: Indiana UP.

Lyotard, Jean-François. 1984. *The Postmodern Condition: A Report on Knowledge*. Minneapolis: U of Minnesota P.

Maddox, J. 1993. "Has Duesberg a Right of Reply?" *Nature* 363: 109.

Maggiore, Christine. 2000. *What If Everything You Thought You Knew about AIDS Was Wrong?* 4th ed. (rev.). Studio City, CA: American Foundation for AIDS Alternatives.

Manjoo, Farhad. 2008. *True Enough: Learning to Live in a Post-Fact Society*. Hoboken, NJ: Wiley.

Mankahlana, P. 2000a. "Building a Monument to Intolerance." Press Release (Mar. 23). Available at www.info.gov.za/speeches/2000/000328927a1001.html.

——. 2000b. "Buying Anti-AIDS Drugs Benefits the Rich." *Business Day*, Mar. 20. Available at www.businessday.co.za/Articles/TarkArticle.aspx?ID=330706.

Manku, M. 2010. "Mehar Manku on Assuming the Editorship of *Medical Hypotheses*." *Medical Hypotheses* 75.3: 275.

Marcus, George. 1999. "Introduction: The Paranoid Style Now." In George Marcus, ed., *Paranoia within Reason: A Casebook on Conspiracy as Explanation*, 1–11. Chicago: U of Chicago P.

Marcuse, Herbert. 1955. *Eros and Civilization*. New York: Vintage.

Martin, B. 2010. "How to Attack a Scientific Theory and Get Away with It (usually): The Attempt to Destroy an Origin-of-AIDS Hypothesis." *Science as Culture* 19.2: 215–39.

Martin, D. 1999. "AZT: A Medicine from Heaven." *The Citizen*, Mar. 31.

Marwick, M. 1964. "Witchcraft as a Social Strain Gauge." *Australian Journal of Science* 26: 263–68.

Mason, Fran. 2002. "A Poor Person's Cognitive Mapping." In Knight, ed., *Conspiracy Nation*, 40–56.

May, M., J. Sterne, D. Costagliola, C. Sabin, A. Phillips, A. Justice, F. Dabis, J. Gill, J. Lundgren, R. Hogg, F. de Wolf, G. Fätkenheuer, S. Staszewski, Monforte A. d'Arminio, and M. Egger. 2006. "HIV Treatment Response and Prognosis in Europe and North America in the First Decade of Highly Active Antiretroviral therapy: A Collaborative Analysis." *The Lancet* 368.9534: 451–58.

Mbali, M. 2004. "AIDS Discourse and the South African State: Government Denialism and Post-Apartheid AIDS Policy Making." *Transformation* 54: 104–122.

Mbeki, Thabo. 1998. "ANC Has No Financial Stake in Virodene." *Mayibuye*hyden (Mar.).

——. 1999. "Address to the National Council of Provinces." Cape Town (Oct. 28). Available at www.anc.org.za/ancdocs/history/mbeki/1999/tm1028.html.

——. 2000a. "Remarks at the First Meeting of the Presidential Advisory Panel on AIDS." Pretoria (May 6). Available at www.anc.org.za/ancdocs/history/mbeki/2000/tm0506.html.

——. 2000b. "Speech at the Opening Session of the 13th International AIDS Conference (July 9). Available at www.anc.org.za/ancdocs/history/mbeki/2000/tm0709.html.

——. 2001. "He Wakened to His Responsibilities": Address by President Thabo Mbeki at the Inaugural ZK Mathews Memorial Lecture, University of Fort Hare (Oct. 12).

Mbeki, Thabo and Peter Mokaba. 2002. "Castro Hlongwane, Caravans, Cats, Geese, Foot and Mouth Statistics: HIV/AIDS and the Struggle for the Humanisation of the African." Unpublished paper, circulated anonymously in the ANC by Peter Mokaba. The document's electronic signature links it to Mbeki—and hence Mbeki is widely believed to be the primary author.

McGregor, Liz. 2009. "Garlic, Olive Oil, Lemons and Beetroot." In Cullinan and Thom, eds., *The Virus, Vitamins and Vegetables*, 130–42.

Melley, T, 2002. "Agency Panic and the Culture of Conspiracy." In Knight, ed., *Conspiracy Nation*, 57–81.

Melville, C. 2009. "Was I Conned by AIDS–AIDS Denialists?" *New Humanist* (Sept.); see http://blog.newhumanist.org.uk/2009/09/was-i-conned-by-aids-denialists.html.

Merton, Robert K. 1957. "The Normative Structure of Science." Reprinted in Helga Nowotny and Klaus Taschwer, eds., *The Sociology of the Sciences*, vol.1 of *The International Library of Critical Writings in Sociology* (1996), 38–49. Cheltenham (Eng.): Edward Elgar.

Miller, H. 2010. "*The Lancet* Pricks Itself." Feb. 5. Available at www.forbes.com/2010/02/05/lancet-vaccines-autism-opinions-contributors-henry-i-miller.html?boxes=Homepagechannels.

Mirowsky, J. and C. Ross. 1983. "Paranoia and the Structure of Powerlessness." *American Sociological Review* 48.2: 228–39.

Montagnier, L. 2002. "A History of HIV Discovery." *Science* 298.5599: 1727–28.

Moore, J. 1996. "Duesberg Adieu!" *Nature* 380: 293–94.

———. 2004. "The Puzzling Origins of AIDS." *American Scientist* 92: 540–47.

Moore, J. and N. Nattrass. 2006. "Deadly Quackery." *New York Times*, June 4.

Mroz, A. 2010. "Decide It on the Science." *Times Higher Education*, Apr. 6. Available at www.timeshighereducation.co.uk/story.asp?sectioncode=26&storycode=411481&c=2.

Msomi, S. and R. Munusamy. 2003. "Manto Wants Aids Dissident as Adviser." *Sunday Times* (South Africa), Mar. 9.

Mtshali, Lionel. 2002. "The War on HIV/AIDS in KwaZulu Natal, State of the Province Speech to the KwaZulu Natal Provincial Legislature" (Feb. 25). Available at www.afrol.com/Countries/South_Africa/documents/mtshali_aids_2002.htm.

Mullis, Kary. 1998. *Dancing Naked in the Mind Field*. New York: Vintage.

Myburgh, J. 2009. "In the Beginning There Was Virodene." In Cullinan and Thom, eds., *The Virus, Vitamins and Vegetables*, 1–15.

Nattrass, N[icoli]. 1994. "Politics and Economics in ANC Economic Policy." *African Affairs* 93: 343–59.

———. 2004. *The Moral Economy of AIDS in South Africa*. Cambridge: Cambridge UP.

———. 2007. *Mortal Combat: AIDS Denialism and the Fight for Antiretrovirals in South Africa*. Pietermaritzburg: U of KwaZulu-Natal P.

———. 2008a. "AIDS and the Scientific Governance of Medicine in Post-Apartheid South Africa." *African Affairs* 107.427: 157–76.

———. 2008b. "Are Country Reputations for Good and Bad AIDS Leadership Deserved? An Exploratory Quantitative Analysis." *Journal of Public Health* 30.4: 398–406.

———. 2009. "Poverty, Sex and HIV." *AIDS and Behavior* 13.5: 833–40.

——. 2011. "Defending the Boundaries of Science: AIDS Denialism, Peer Review and the *Medical Hypotheses* Saga." *Sociology of Health and Illness*. Published online (DOI: 10.1111/j.1467–9566.2010.01312.x) on Feb. 11. Available at http://online library.wiley.com/doi/10.1111/j.1467–9566.2010.01312.x/full.

Nattrass, N. and J. Bergman. 2007. "La creciente amenaza de los que niegan el sida." *Actualizaciones en Sida* 15.57 (Sept.): 106–114.

Nattrass, N. and N. Geffen. 2005. "The Impact of Reduced Drug Prices on the Cost-Effectiveness of HAART in South Africa." *African Journal of AIDS Research* 4.1: 65–67.

Navario, Peter. 2009. "Implementation of a Novel Model to Boost Routine HIV Care and Treatment Capacity in South Africa: Outcomes, Costs, and Cost-Effectiveness." PhD diss., University of Cape Town, Cape Town.

Ndebele, N. 2004. "The Dilemmas of Leadership: HIV/AIDS and the State Consolidation in South Africa." In M. Chabani, ed., *On Becoming a Democracy: Transition and Transformation*. Pretoria: UNISA Press.

Ndung'u, T., E. Sepako, M. McLane, F. Chand, K. Bedi, S. Gaseitsiwe, F. Doualla-Bell, T. Peter, I. Thior, S. Moyo, P. Gilbert, V. Novitsky, and M. Essex. 2006. "HIV-1 Subtype C In Vitro Growth and Coreceptor Utilization." *Virology* 347: 247–60.

Niehaus, I. and G. Jonsson. 2005. "Dr. Wouter Basson, Americans, and Wild Beasts: Men's Conspiracy Theories of HIV/AIDS in the South African Lowveld." *Medical Anthropology* 24.2: 179–208.

Nolan, Stephanie. 2007. *28 Stories of AIDS in Africa*. London: Portobello Books.

Nyhan, B. and J. Reifler. 2010. "When Corrections Fail: The Persistence of Political Misperceptions." *Political Behavior* 32: 303–330.

O'Brien, S. and J. Goedert. 1996. "HIV Causes AIDS: Koch's Postulates Fulfilled." *Current Opinion in Immunology* 8: 613–18.

Offit, Paul. 2008. *Autism's False Prophets: Bad Science, Risky Medicine, and the Search for a Cure*. New York: Columbia UP.

Ornstein, C., Costello, D. 2005. "A Mother's Denial, a Daughter's Death." *Los Angeles Times*, Sept. 24.

Owen, R., J. Heitman, D. Hirschkorn, M. Lanteri, H. Biswas, J. Martin, M. Krone, S. Norris, and J. Philip. 2010. "HIV+ Elite Controllers Have Low HIV-specific T-cell Activation Yet Maintain Strong, Polyfunctional T-cell Responses." *AIDS* 24.8: 1095–1105.

Paglia C. 2003. *"Cults and Cosmic Consciousness: Religious Vision in the American 1960s." Arion* 10.3: 57–111.

Palella, F., K. Delaney, A. Moorman, M. Loveless, J. Fuhrer, G. Satten, D. Aschman, and S. Holmberg. 1998. "Declining Morbidity and Mortality among Patients with Advanced Human Immunodeficiency Virus Infection." *New England Journal of Medicine* 338.13: 853–60.

Papadopulos-Eleopulos, E., V. Turner, J. Papadimitriou, D. Causer, A. Hellman, and T. Miller. 1999. "A Critical Analysis of the Pharmacology of AZT and Its Use in AIDS." *Current Medical Research and Opinion* 15 (Supp. 1): s1–45.

Parsons, S., W. Simmons, F. Shinhoster, and J. Kilburn. 1999. "A Test of the Grape-Vine: An Empirical Examination of Conspiracy Theories among African Americans." *Sociological Spectrum* 19: 201–222.

Partridge, C. H. 2005. *The Re-enchantment of the West: Alternative Spiritualities, Sacralization, Popular Culture, and Occulture.* London and New York: T. & T. Clark.

Phillips, Howard. 2004. "HIV AIDS in the Context of South Africa's Epidemic History." In Kauffman and Lindauer, eds., *AIDS and South Africa*, 31–47.

Picardie, J. 2002. "MMR: Who to Believe, the Whistleblower, the Medical Establishment and the Parents Put Their Case." *The Telegraph*, June 8.

Pipes, Daniel. 1997. *Conspiracy.* New York: The Free Press.

Posel, D., K. Kahn, and L. Walker. 2007. "Living with Death in a Time of AIDS: A Rural South African Case Study." *Scandinavian Journal of Public Health* 35 (Supp. 69): 138–46.

Presidential AIDS Advisory Panel Report (PAAPR). 2001. *Presidential AIDS Advisory Panel Report: A Synthesis Report of the deliberations by the panel of experts invited by the President of the Republic of South Africa, the Honourable Thabo Mbeki.* This report is available at www.info.gov.za/otherdocs/2001/aidspanelpdf.pdf.

Price, D. 2007a. "Buying a Piece of Anthropology. Part 1: Human Ecology and Unwitting Anthropological Research for the CIA." *Anthropology Today* 23.3: 8–13.

———. 2007b. "Buying a Piece of Anthropology. Part 2: The CIA and Our Tortured Past." *Anthropology Today* 23.5: 17–22.

Räikkä, J. "On Political Conspiracy Theories." *The Journal of Philosophy* 17.2: 185–201.

Rasnick, D. 2000. Talked with President Thabo Mbeki. Unpublished piece available at www.virusmyth.com/aids/news/drtalkmbeki.htm.

Reverby, S. 2009. *Examining Tuskegee: The Infamous Syphilis Study and Its Legacy.* Chapel Hill: U of North Carolina P.

———. 2011. "Normal Exposure and Inoculation Syphilis: A PHS 'Tuskegee' Doctor in Guatemala, 1946–48." *Journal of Policy History* 23: 6–28.

Richman, D. et al. 1987. "The Toxicity of Azidothymidine (AZT) in the Treatment of Patients with AIDS and AIDS-related Complex: A Double-blind, Placebo-controlled Trial." *New England Journal of Medicine* 317: 192–97.

Richman, D., D. Margolis, M. Delaney, W. Greene, D. Hazuda, and R. Pomeranz. 2009. "The Challenge of Finding a Cure for HIV Infection." *Science* 323.5019: 1304–1307.

Roberts, J. 1992. "About Turn in US on Interferon Alpha." *British Medical Journal* 305: 1243–44.

Rödlach, Alexander. 2006. *Witches, Westerners, and HIV: AIDS and Cultures of Blame in Africa.* Walnut Creek, CA: Left Coast Press.

Rosen, S., B. Larson, A. Brennan, L. Long, M. Fox, C. Mongwenyana, M. Ketlkhapile, and I. Sanne. 2010. "Economic Outcomes of Patients Receiving Antiretroviral Therapy for HIV/AIDS in South Africa Are Sustained Through Three years on Treatment." *PLoS ONE* 5.1: 1–8.

Ross, M., J. Essien, and I. Torres. 2006. "Conspiracy Beliefs about the Origin of HIV/AIDS in Four Racial Groups." *Journal of Acquired Immune Deficiency Syndromes* 41.3: 342–44.

Rubincam, C. 2008. *Managing Conspiracy Theories in Public Health: Ensuring That Voice Does Not Lead to Exit.* Development Studies Institute, London School of Economics and Political Science. Working Paper No. 08–88.

Rybicki, E., A. Williamson, and L. Morris. 2000. "AIDS Denialists Aren't Victims—But the People Their Ideas Kill Will Be." *Nature* 405: 273.

Sabatier, Renée. 1988. *Blaming Others: Prejudice, Race, and Worldwide AIDS.* Washington, D.C.: The Panos Institute.

Sanders, T. and H. West. 2003. "Power Revealed and Concealed in the New World Order." In Sanders and West, eds., *Transparency and Conspiracy*, 1–37.

Sanders, Todd and Harry West, eds. *Transparency and Conspiracy: Ethnographies of Suspicion in the New World Order.* Durham, NC: Duke UP.

Sawers, L. and E. Stillwaggon. 2010. "Understanding the Southern African 'Anomoly': Poverty, Endemic Disease and HIV." *Development and Change* 41.2: 195–224.

Schmidt, C. 2008. "Profile: Vera Sharav" *Nature Biotechnology* 26: 965.

Schneider, H. 2002. "On the Fault Line: The Politics of AIDS Policy in Contemporary South Africa." *African Studies* 612.1: 145–67.

Schneider, H. and D. Fassin. 2002. "Denial and Defiance: A Socio-Political Analysis of AIDS in South Africa." *AIDS* 16: s45–s51.

Schüklenk, U. 2004. "Professional Responsibilities of Biomedical Scientists in Public Discourse." *Journal of Medical Ethics* 30: 53–60.

Scott, J. and L. Kaufman. 2005. "Belated Charges Ignites Furor over AIDS Drug Trial," *New York Times*, July 17.

Sedgwick, Mark. 2004. *Against the Modern World: Traditionalism and the Secret Intellectual History of the Twentieth Century.* Oxford: Oxford UP.

Shabazz, S. 2004. "Activists Charge Pharmaceutical Cartel with Being a Tool for Genocide." *Final Call* (Jan 20); see www.finalcall.com/artman/publish/National_News_2/Activists_charge_pharmaceutical_cartel_with_being__1247.shtml.

Shaffer, M. 2001. "Officers Kill Militia Voice, Deputy Shot." *Arizona Republic*, Nov. 7; see www.rickross.com/reference/militia/militia53.html.

Shaffer, N., R. Chuachoowong, P. Mock, C. Bhadrakom, W. Siniwisin, N. Young, T. Chotpitayasunndh, S. Chearskul, A. Roongpisuthipong, P. Chinayon, J. Karon, D. Mastro, and R. Simons on behalf of the Bangkok Collaborative Perinatal HIV Transmission Study Group. 1999. "Short-course Zidovudine for Perinatal HIV-1 Transmission in Bangkok, Thailand: A Randomised Clinical Trial." *The Lancet* 353: 773–80.

Sharp, P. and B. Hahn. 2010. The evolution of HIV-1 and the origin of AIDS. *Philosophical Transactions of the Royal Society* 365: 2487–94.

Sheckels, T. 2004. "The Rhetoric of Thabo Mbeki on HIV/Aids: Strategic Scapegoating." *Harvard Journal of Communication* 15: 69–82.

Shenton, Joan. 2000. "Sitting Down with President Mbeki" (interview). Aired on *Carte Blanche* (Apr. 16). Available at www.virusmyth.com/aids/news/jsinter viewmbeki.htm.

Showalter, Elaine. 1997. *Hystories: Hysterical Epidemics and Modern Culture*. New York: Columbia UP.

Siahpush M. 1998. "Post-modern Values, Dissatisfaction with Conventional Medicine and Popularity of Alternative Therapies." *Journal of Sociology 34.1:* 58–70.

Simmons, W. and S. Parsons. 2005. "Beliefs in Conspiracy Theories Among African Americans: A Comparison of Elites and Masses." *Social Science Quarterly* 86.3: 582–98.

Singh, Robert. 1997. *The Farrakhan Phenomenon: Race, Reaction, and the Paranoid Style in American Politics*. Washington, D.C.: Georgetown UP.

Smit, G., R. Geskus, S. Walker, C. Sabin, R. Couthino, K. Porter, M. Prins, and the CASCADE Collaboration. 2006. "Effective Therapy Has Altered the Spectrum of Cause-Specific Mortality Following HIV Serocoversion." *AIDS* 20.50: 741–49.

Smith, R. 2005. "Medical Journals Are an Extension of the Marketing Arm of Pharmaceutical Companies." *PLoS Med* 2.5: e138. Published online (DOI: 10.1371/journal.pmed.0020138).

Smith, T. and S. Novella. 2007. "HIV Denial in the Internet Era." *PLoS Medicine* 4.8: e256. Published online (DOI: 10.1371/journal.pmed.0040256).

Sonnabend, J. 2000. "Honoring with Pride 2000 Honoree: Joseph Sonnabend." Comment published in connection with the AmfAR award. Available at www. amfar.org/spotlight/article.aspx?id=4550.

Sparks, Allister. 2003. *Beyond the Miracle: Inside the New South Africa*. Chicago: U of Chicago P.

Spaulding, A., B. Stephenson, G. Macalino, W. Ruby, J. Clarke, and T. Flanigan. 2002. "Human Immunodeficiency Virus in Correctional Facilities: A Review." *Clinical Infectious Diseases* 35.3: 305–312.

Specter, Michael. 2010. *Denialism: How Irrational Thinking Hinders Scientific Progress, Harms the Planet and Threatens Our Lives*. London: Penguin.

Stadler, J. 2003. "Rumor, Gossip and Blame: Implications for HIV/AIDS Prevention in the South African Lowveld." *AIDS Education and Prevention* 15.4: 357–68.

Steinberg, J[onny]. 2007. "Anthropology of Low Expectations." *Business Day*, June 5; see http://allafrica.com/stories/200706050338.

——. 2008. *Three-letter Plague*. Cape Town: Jonathan Ball.

Stewart. G. (et al.). 2000. "The Durban Declaration Is Not Accepted by All." *Nature* 407: 286. The letter was also signed by S. Mhlongo, E. De Harven, C. Fiala, C. Kohnlein, A. Herxheimer, P. Duesberg, D. Rasnick, R. Giraldo, M. Kothari, H. Bialy, and C. Gesheckter.

Strine, T., R. Kobau, D. Chapman, D. Thurman, P. Price, and L. Ballus. 2005. "Psychological Distress, Comorbidities, and Health Behaviours among US Adults with Seizures: Results from the 2002 National Health Interview Survey." *Epilepsia* 46.7: 1133–39.

Suls, J. and R. Martin. 2009. "The Air We Breathe: A Critical Look at Practices and Altermatives in the Peer-review Process." *Perspectives on Psychological Science* 4.1: 40–50.

Thom, A. 2009. "The Curious Tale of the Vitamin Seller." In Cullinan and Thom, eds., *The Virus, Vitamins and Vegetables*, 112–29.

Thomas, K., J. Nicholl, and P. Coleman. 2001. "Use and Expenditure on Complementary Medicine in England: A Population-Based Survey." *Complementary Therapies in Medicine* 9.1: 2–11.

Thomas, S. and S. Quinn. 1991. "The Tuskegee Syphilis Study, 1932 to 1972: Implications for HIV Education and AIDS Risk Education Programs in the Black Community." *American Journal of Public Health* 81.11: 1498–1505.

——. 1993. "The Burdens of Race and History on Black Americans' Attitudes Toward Needle Exchange Policy to Prevent HIV Disease." *Journal of Public Health Policy* 14.3: 320–47.

Thompson, Damien. 2008. *Counterknowledge: How We Surrendered to Conspiracy Theories, Quack Medicine, Bogus Science and Fake History*. London: Atlantic Books.

Tindle, H., R. Davis, R. Phillips, and D. Eisenberg. 2005. "Trends in the Use of Complementary and Alternative Medicine by US Adults: 1997–2002." *Alternative Therapies in Health and Medicine* 11.1: 42–49.

Trafimow, D. and S. Rice. 2009. "What If Social Scientists Had Reviewed Great Scientific Works of the Past?" *Perspectives on Psychological Science* 4.1: 65–78.

Treichler, Paula. 1999. *How to Have Theory in an Epidemic: Cultural Chronicles of AIDS*. Durham (NC) and London: Duke UP.

Tun, W., S. Kellerman, S. Maime et al. 2010. Conspiracy beliefs about HIV, attitudes towards condoms and treatment and HIV-related preventive behaviors among men who have sex with men in Tshwane (Pretoria), South Africa. 18th International AIDS Conference, Vienna (abstract TUPE0656).

Turner, Patricia. 1994. *I Heard It Through the Grapevine: Rumor in African-American Culture*. Berkeley: U of California P.

Turner, V. 2006. Affidavit (in the Andre Parenzee case, Australia). Available at http://garlan.org/Cases/Parenzee/Turner-Affidavit.pdf.

UNAIDS. 2010. *Outlook Report*, UNAIDS, Geneva. Available at http://data.un aids.org/pub/Outlook/2010/20100713_outlook_report_web_en.pdf.

US Department of State. 1987. "The USSR's AIDS Disinformation Campaign." In *Foreign Affairs Note* (July). US Department of State, Washington, D.C.

Van der Vliet, Virginia. 2004. "South Africa Divided Against AIDS: A Crisis of Leadership." In Kauffman and Lindauer, eds., *AIDS and South Africa*, 48–96.

Van Heuverswyn, F. and M. Peeters. 2007. "The Origins of HIV and Implications for the Global epidemic." *Current Infectious Disease Reports* 9: 338–46.

Volberding, P. and S. Deeks. 2010. "Antiretroviral Therapy and Management of HIV Infection." *The Lancet* 376: 49–62.

Volmink, Jimmy, Nandi Siegfried, Lize van der Merwe, and Peter Brocklehurst. 2007. "Antiretrovirals for Reducing the Risk of Mother to Child Transmission of HIV Infection." In *Cochrane Database of Systematic Reviews* 1. Art. No. CD003510. Published online (DOI: 10.1002/145651858/CD003510.pub2).

Wakefield, A., M. Blaxill, B. Haley, A. Ryland, D. Hollenbeck, J. Johnson, J. Moody, and C. Stott. 2009. "Response to Dr. Ari Brown and the Immunization Action Coalition." *Medical Veritas* 6: 1907–1924. Available at www.medicalveritas.com/manWakefield.pdf.

Wakefield, A., S. Murch, A. Anthony, J. Linnell, D. Casson, M. Malik, M. Berelowitz, A. Dhillon, M. Thomson, P. Harvey, A. Valentine, S. Davies, and J. Walker-Smith. 1998. "Ileal-Lymphoid-Nodular Hyperplasia, Non-specific Colitis, and Pervasive Developmental Disorder in Children." *The Lancet* 532: 637–41.

Wakefield, J. 1997. "Trial and Error." *Washington City Paper*, Apr. 11; see www.washingtoncitypaper.com/articles/12439/trial-and-error/.

Wang, J. 2008. "AIDS Denialism and the 'Humanisation of the African,'" *Race and Class* 41.3: 1–18.

Weinel, M. 2007. "Primary Source Knowledge and Technical Decision-Making: Mbeki and the AZT Debate: Part A." *Studies in History and Philosophy of Science* 38.4: 748–60.

——. 2008. "Counterfeit Scientific Controversies in Science Policy Contexts." In Cardiff School of Social Science, Paper No. 120 (Nov.).

———. 2009. "Thabo Mbeki, HIV/AIDS and Bogus Scientific Controversies." Available at www.politicsweb.co.za/politicsweb/view/politicsweb/en/page71619 ?oid=121968&sn=Detail.

———. 2010. "Technological Decision-making Under Scientific Uncertainty: Preventing Mother-to-Child Transmission of HIV in South Africa." PhD diss., Cardiff University (Dec.).

Weiss, R. and H. Jaffe. 1990. "Duesberg, HIV and AIDS." *Nature* 345: 659–60.

Weller, Ann. 2001. *Editorial Peer-review: Its Strengths and Weaknesses.* Washington, D.C.: ASIST and Thomas Hogan.

Whetten, K., J. Leserman, R. Whetten, J. Ostermann, N. Theilman, M. Swartz, and D. Stangle. 2006. "Exploring Lack of Trust in Care Providers and the Government as a Barrier to Health Service Use." *American Journal of Public Health* 96: 716–21. Published online (DOI: 10.2105/*AJPH*.2005.063255).

Whitfield, L. 2000a. "Bite the Bullet." *POZ* (July); see www.poz.com/articles/ 203_10295.shtml.

———. 2000b. "The Secret Plot to Destroy African Americans." *POZ* (Dec.); see www.poz.com/articles/208_7602.shtml.

Willman, Skip. 2002. "Spinning Paranoia: The Ideologies of Conspiracy and Contingency in Postmodern Culture." In Knight, ed., *Conspiracy Nation*, 21–39.

Willsher, K. 1999. "To poor blacks, heart surgeon Dr Wouter Basson is a saviour. Could he also have been apartheid's poisoner-in-chief, murdering 229 black activists with cyanide chocolates, umbrella tips . . . and even toxic underpants?" *Mail on Sunday* (London), May 23.

Wilson, M. 1951. "Witch Beliefs and Social Structure." *American Journal of Sociology* 56.4: 307–313.

Wittes, B. 1993. "Miracle Worker?" *Washington City Paper*, Sept. 3; see www.wash ingtoncitypaper.com/articles/8414/miracle-worker.

World Health Organization (WHO). 2000. *Safety and Tolerability of Zidovudine.* Available at www.who.int/reproductive-health/docs/zidovudine.htm.

———. 2003. "Antiretroviral Therapy in Primary Health Care: Experience of the Khayelitsha Programme in South Africa." Case Study: Perspectives and Practice in Antiretroviral Treatment. Available at www.who.int/hiv/amds/case8.pdf.

Worobey, M., M. Gemmel, D. Teuwen, T. Haselkorn, Kl Kunstman, M. Brunce, J. Muyembe, J. Kabongo, R. Kalengayi, E. van Marck, T. Gilbert, and S. Wolinksy. 2008. "Direct Evidence of Extensive Diversity of HIV-1 in Kinshasa by 1960." *Nature* 455: 661–64.

Worobey, M., M. Santiago, B. Keele, J. Ndkango, J. Joy, B. Labama, B. Dheda, A. Rambaut, P. Sharp, G. Shaw, and B. Hahn. 2004. "Origin of AIDS: Contaminated Polio Vaccine Theory Refuted." *Nature* 428: 820.

Youde, Jeremy. 2007. *AIDS, South Africa and the Politics of Knowledge*. Ashgate (Hampshire, UK): Aldershot.

Ziman, John. 1966. *Public Knowledge: The Social Dimension of Science*. Cambridge: Cambridge UP.

Zuckerman, H. and R. Merton. 1971. "Patterns of Evaluation in Science: Institutionalisation, Structure and Functions of the Referee System." *Minerva* 9.1: 66–100.

INDEX